MW01345763

Sign Language Processing

Achraf Othman

Sign Language Processing

From Gesture to Meaning

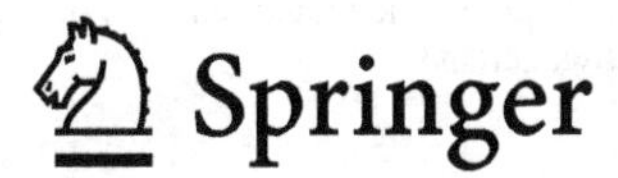

Achraf Othman
Mada Qatar Assistive Technology Center
Doha, Qatar

ISBN 978-3-031-68762-4 ISBN 978-3-031-68763-1 (eBook)
https://doi.org/10.1007/978-3-031-68763-1

This Springer imprint is published by the registered company Springer Nature Switzerland AG
The registered company address is: Gewerbestrasse 11, 6330 Cham, Switzerland

For Father and Mother
For Marwa
For Maram & Jumana

Preface

The idea for this book took root during a conversation with a close friend who was deaf in 2006. He was asking if mobile phones could facilitate their communication. As we communicated through a mix of sign language and written messages, I was struck by the beauty, expressiveness, and complexity of sign language. This realization sparked a desire to dive deeper into the world of visual-spatial languages, to understand their intricacies, and to explore the technologies that could enhance communication and accessibility for deaf and hard-of-hearing individuals.

In 2008, I got the opportunity to join Jemni's Lab, UTIC, at the University of Tunis to start working on a project called SportSign. This project aims to provide live sports news for the deaf community in Tunisia through an avatar broadcasted in the Multimedia Message Service (MMS). The work was presented during ICCHP 2010 and published in Lecture Notes of Computer Science by Springer.[1] This was the actual start in my career to address challenges encountered by the deaf.

Sign Language Processing is the culmination of years of research, collaboration, and passion. It is intended to serve as a comprehensive resource for linguists, educators, researchers, technology enthusiasts, and anyone interested in sign languages and their applications in the modern world.

In writing this book, I sought to bridge the gap between the linguistic aspects of sign languages and the ever-evolving landscape of technology. Understanding the unique characteristics and structure of sign languages is essential for developing effective technologies that can truly make a difference in the lives of deaf and hard-of-hearing individuals.

Throughout the writing process, I was fortunate to collaborate with numerous experts in linguistics, education, computer science, and artificial intelligence. Their invaluable contributions have greatly enriched the content of this book, ensuring

[1]Othman, A., El Ghoul, O., Jemni, M. (2010). SportSign: A Service to Make Sports News Accessible to Deaf Persons in Sign Languages. In: Miesenberger, K., Klaus, J., Zagler, W., Karshmer, A. (eds) Computers Helping People with Special Needs. ICCHP 2010. Lecture Notes in Computer Science, vol 6180. Springer, Berlin, Heidelberg. https://doi.org/10.1007/978-3-642-14100-3_26

that it offers a well-rounded, interdisciplinary perspective on sign language processing.

While the book covers a wide array of topics, from the history of sign languages to the latest technological advancements, it is essential to note that the field of sign language processing is continuously evolving. As such, this book should be seen as a snapshot of the current state of the art, with the understanding that breakthroughs and developments will continue to shape the field.

I sincerely hope this book will inspire curiosity, foster understanding, and contribute to the ongoing dialogue surrounding sign languages and their place in our increasingly interconnected world. I aim to see the power of technology harnessed to enhance communication, accessibility, and inclusion for deaf and hard-of-hearing individuals, promoting a more equitable and diverse society.

I am deeply grateful to all who have supported and contributed to this project, and I am excited to share *Sign Language Processing* with readers worldwide.

Writing a book always involves more people than just me. I extend my most profound appreciation to Maha Al Mansouri and Amani Al Tamimi, from Mada Qatar Assistive Technology Center, for their unlimited support. I am also indebted to the diligent teams at the Mada and the accessibility team of the LaTICE research laboratory at the University of Tunis, whose feedback enriched our perspectives.

Undoubtedly, Prof. Mohamed Jemni's guidance since 2007 has been a beacon, and his expertise is a foundation to which I owe immense respect and admiration. The project I was involved in, WebSign, was an inspiration for all team members.

Special thanks go to Dr. Sameer Samreen, the sign language interpreter and Expert at Al Jazeera Channel, for providing advice and media content to understand the sign language structure well.

Doha, Qatar Achraf Othman

About the Book

This book is a comprehensive exploration of the fascinating world of sign languages and the innovative technologies designed to enhance communication and accessibility for deaf and hard-of-hearing individuals. This book is the result of extensive research, collaboration, and dedication, aiming to raise awareness, foster understanding, and promote the development of tools and resources to bridge communication gaps.

The book is organized into several chapters, each focusing on a specific aspect of sign languages, their structure, the technologies employed in their processing, and the broader societal implications of these advancements. Readers are introduced to sign languages' foundations, history, importance, and unique features that distinguish them from spoken languages. The book then looks into the complex structure of sign languages, covering phonology, morphology, syntax, semantics, and pragmatics.

The world is home to a diverse array of sign languages, and the book highlights a selection of these, including American, Arabic, French, and International Sign Languages, as well as regional and indigenous varieties. The role of deaf communities in shaping the evolution and development of these languages is emphasized, showcasing the richness and vitality of sign language communication.

The book also addresses sign language acquisition and education, discussing first and second language acquisition, teaching and learning strategies, and the role of technology in sign language education. This provides valuable insights for educators, learners, and researchers alike.

The book's central focus is sign language processing, covering a range of topics, including natural language processing, gesture recognition, motion tracking technologies, and machine learning approaches. The challenges and limitations inherent in these fields are discussed, offering a balanced and informed perspective on the current state of sign language processing technology.

Machine translation techniques for sign languages are explored in depth, with chapters on statistical and neural machine translation, as well as the challenges, limitations, and ethical considerations surrounding these methods. Additionally, the book investigates the development and deployment of avatars for sign language interpretation and the various technologies designed to improve accessibility for deaf and hard-of-hearing individuals.

Lastly, the broader societal impact of sign language processing is examined, touching on digital accessibility in education and the workplace, the role of sign language processing in bridging communication gaps, the empowerment of deaf communities through technology, and the legal and policy implications of these advancements.

Contents

About the Author

Achraf Othman specializes in sign language processing, digital accessibility, the accessible Metaverse, and artificial intelligence for education, having been dedicated to the field since 2007. He earned his M.Sc. in Computer Science from the Higher National Engineering School of Tunis at the University of Tunis (ex ESSTT) and furthered his expertise with a Ph.D. from the University of Sfax, Tunisia.

Since 2010, Dr. Othman has taught Computer Science as Assistant Professor at two universities. Throughout his academic journey, he has shared his knowledge on subjects ranging from operating systems and programming to computer vision. Recently, he joined Hamad Bin Khalifa University as an adjunct assistant professor.

He has mentored numerous bachelor's and master's students, guiding them to academic success. In addition to his teaching, Dr. Othman is affiliated as a researcher with the Research Laboratory LaTICE at the University of Tunis.

Currently, he is the Head of the Innovation and Research Section at the Mada Qatar Assistive Technology Center in Doha, Qatar. Here, he investigates IT industry challenges, particularly in assistive technology and digital accessibility. Dr. Othman leads projects that leverage cutting-edge technologies, natural language processing, and artificial intelligence to develop solutions that empower individuals with disabilities.

Questions or comments?

Email at contact@achrafothman.net or visit website at www.achrafothman.net

Abbreviations

AI	Artificial Intelligence
AIB	Agglomerative Information Bottleneck
ArSL	Arab Sign Language Family
ASL	American Sign Language
ASLLVD	American Sign Language Lexicon Video Dataset
BASL	Black American Sign Language (an ASL dialect)
BI-BI	Bilingual-Bicultural
BSL	British Sign Language
CL	Classifier
CNN	Convolutional Neural Networks
CSL	Chinese Sign Language
DBSCAN	Density-Based Spatial Clustering of Applications with Noise
DSL	Danish Sign Language
EMG	Electromyography
FAR	False Accept Rate
GCN	Graph Convolutional Networks
GRU	Gated Recurrent Units
GSL	Ghanaian Sign Language
HamNoSys	Hamburg Notation System
HMM	Hidden Markov Models
IPSL	Indo-Pakistani Sign Language
IS	International Sign
IoU	Intersection over Union
JSL	Japanese Sign Language
KSL	Kazakh Sign Language (an RSL Dialect)
Libras	Brazilian Sign Language
LIS	Italian Sign Language (in Italian: *Lingua dei Segni Italiana*)
LSF	French Sign Language (in French: *Langue des Signes Française*)
LSQ	Quebec Sign Language (in French: *Langue des signes Québécoise*)
LSTM	Long Short-Term Memory Networks
ML	Machine Learning

MSE	Mean Squared Error
MT	Machine Translation
NGT	Dutch Sign Language (in Dutch: *Nederlandse Gebarentaal*)
NLP	Natural Language Processing
NZSL	New Zealand Sign Language
QSL	Qatari Sign Language
RID	Registry of Interpreters for the Deaf
RSL	Russian Sign Language
SASL	South African Sign Language
SCD	Skin Color Detection
SL	Sign Language
SLNS	Sign Language Notation System
SLP	Sign Language Processing
SLR	Sign Language Recognition
SLT	Sign Language Translation
SOM	Self-Organizing Maps
SSL	Swedish Sign Language
SVM	Support Vector Machines
TASL	Tactile ASL
TSL	Taiwan Sign Language
UG	Universal Grammar
VGT	Flemish Sign Language (in Dutch: *Vlaamse Gebarentaal*)
WHO	World Health Organization
WLASL	Word-Level American Sign Language

Chapter 1
Preamble

1.1 Introduction

Within the vast domain of human communication, specific modes of expression, including sign and visual-spatial languages, are notably captivating and profoundly singular. The ubiquity of speech across cultures has marginalized these modes, relegating them to specialized discussion domains [1]. Nonetheless, the significance and pertinence of these matters cannot be emphasized sufficiently. In addition to serving as a mode of communication, sign languages are deeply ingrained cultural and identity indicators for deaf and hard-of-hearing communities [2]. These languages provide linguists and researchers with a singular opportunity to investigate human cognition's extraordinary versatility and adaptability and the profound depths of information processing and transmission that can be attained without vocal speech [3].

Verbal communication predominantly depends on auditory and vocal modalities. By contrast, sign and visual-spatial languages utilize the potential of spatiality to construct narratives and mental images through spatial configurations and gestures [4]. The distinction between spoken and sign languages extends beyond their modes of communication and comprises many additional facets. Sign languages are distinguished by their grammatical systems, inherent structures, and cultural nuances, making their study challenging and rewarding [5].

Although visual-spatial languages are communication systems that depend significantly on visual and spatial cues, their linguistic complexity is lower than sign languages. As assistance systems, visual-spatial languages like Makaton [6] and Cued Speech [7] are frequently implemented for those who have hearing impairments. Physical signals, facial expressions, and gestures facilitate communication and comprehension. In contrast, the grammatical, syntactic, and lexical aspects of sign languages, including American Sign Language (ASL), British Sign Language (BSL), and French Sign Language (LSF), have been developed. They have

A. Othman, *Sign Language Processing*,
https://doi.org/10.1007/978-3-031-68763-1_1

developed organically over time and are predominantly utilized by communities of deaf individuals in the United States, United Kingdom, and France [8].

The tenacity of the deaf community is celebrated throughout the development of visual-spatial and sign languages. These languages, which originated from necessity and developed within tightly bonded communities, have significantly impacted the identity and culture of deaf communities worldwide [9]. The development of these languages is documented as a series of challenges, accomplishments, and, ultimately, success. The examination of visual-spatial languages further complicates their investigation. In contrast to conventional sign languages, visual-spatial languages challenge preconceived conceptions regarding language formation, structure, and comprehension. The distinctive characteristics of these languages include intriguing challenges for linguists and technologists [10].

This chapter explores these languages, beginning with their definitions and concluding with their extensive ramifications on technology and society. This investigation will serve as a foundation for subsequent chapters, equipping readers with the essential understanding required to fully comprehend visual and spatial language's complex intricacies and subtleties.

1.2 Hard-of-Hearing and Deafness

According to the World Health Organization, hearing difficulties and deafness affect a significant portion of the global population [11]. These conditions affect individuals' ability to perceive and understand sounds, which can profoundly affect their daily lives. Hearing loss may range from mild to severe for individuals who are difficult to hear, making it challenging to comprehend speech or other auditory cues [12].

Globally, hearing impairment is a significant public health concern, as the staggering statistics show that over 1.5 billion individuals are affected by hearing loss in at least one ear.[1] Approximately 430 million people experience hearing loss, necessitating rehabilitation services to aid them daily [13]. Even with technological interventions such as hearing aids, approximately 13% of adults aged 18 years and older still report difficulties in hearing, indicating that current solutions do not fully address the challenges encountered. This issue becomes more pronounced with age; data show that over 14% of adults aged >65 years rely on hearing aids [14]. The situation is projected to escalate, with estimates indicating that by 2050, approximately 700 million people will have disabling hearing loss [15], highlighting the urgent need for comprehensive strategies to manage and mitigate hearing impairment on a global scale [16].

According to a recent survey conducted by OnePoll for Forbes Health involving 500 U.S. adults with hearing loss, the results reveal diverse perceptions about the

[1] Forbes: https://www.forbes.com/health/hearing-aids/deafness-statistics/

causes of their condition. Over half of the respondents attribute their hearing loss to aging or natural causes, commonly called presbycusis [17]. Conversely, another segment comprising approximately 50% of the participants believes their hearing loss may be linked to side effects associated with their medications. Additionally, 48% of those surveyed reported hearing loss due to exposure to loud noises at their workplace, while 43% associated it with injuries (refer to Table 1.1 for detailed statistics).

Communication can significantly challenge individuals with hearing impairment or deafness. Beyond the inability to perceive and understand sounds, these conditions can affect an individual's ability to communicate effectively verbally. Those with mild hearing loss may struggle to follow conversations, particularly in noisy environments. In contrast, those with severe hearing loss or deafness may rely on alternative communication methods, such as visual-spatial and sign language or lip-reading.

Figure 1.1, a photo of Cottonbro Studio from Pexels, captures a communicative exchange between a man and a young female counterpart, utilizing sign language as the medium of interaction. The temporality of the photograph is situated within the COVID-19 pandemic epoch,[2] when wearing masks was mandated as a public health measure. Notably, the image features a service provider providing a transparent face covering, a deliberate modification to the traditional mask that preserves the visibility of facial expressions, an integral component of sign language communication. The photograph is an illustrative artifact that sheds light on the intersection of public health directives and the consequential modifications necessary for deaf and hard-of-hearing communities. The transparent mask emerges as a symbolic embodiment of inclusivity, ensuring that communication barriers are mitigated and highlighting the importance of the facial expression channel in sign language.

The impact of hearing and deafness on communication extends beyond spoken language. It can also affect an individual's ability to engage in social interactions, educational settings, and professional environments. The need for accommodations,

Table 1.1 Causes of hearing loss

	Hearing loss level			
Causes	Mild	Moderate	Severe	Profound
Accident/injury	45	46	45	19
Disease symptoms and side effects	52	38	36	38
Exposure to deafening noise at work/in a professional setting	44	53	50	44
Exposure to deafening noise in a recreational setting	37	25	29	38
Genetic factors	19	11	19	19
Medication side effects	57	56	36	31
Natural causes/aging	56	54	62	44

[2] Information about COVID-19: https://www.who.int/emergencies/diseases/novel-coronavirus-2019/question-and-answers-hub/q-a-detail/coronavirus-disease-covid-19

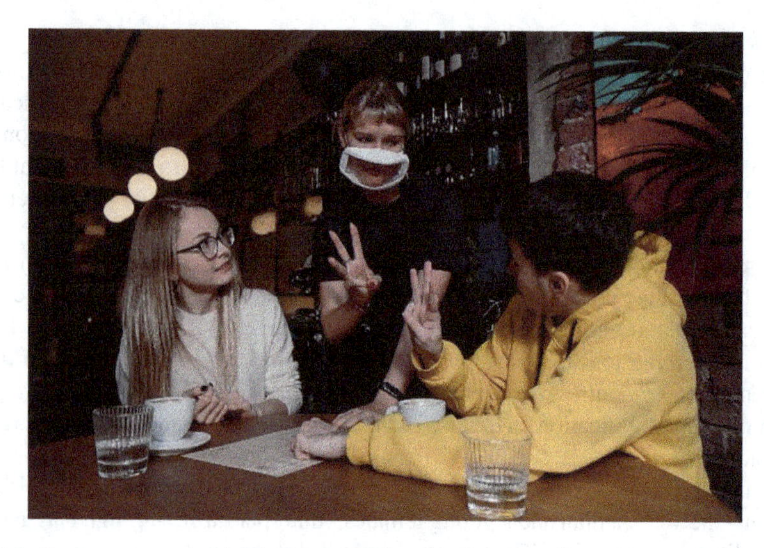

Fig. 1.1 Persons communicating in Sign Language (Credit to Photo by cottonbro studio: https://www.pexels.com/photo/man-in-yellow-hoodie-jacket-ordering-to-a-waitress-through-sign-language-6322051/)

such as captioning, sign language interpreters, or hearing aids, is crucial for facilitating effective communication among individuals with these conditions.

Visual-spatial and sign languages are paramount in facilitating communication among deaf individuals because they offer a visual means of expression through hand gestures, facial expressions, and body language. Such language enables deaf individuals to express themselves, comprehend others, and interact significantly. Consequently, the primary challenge is identifying effective communication systems that address these unique requirements.

Deaf individuals often form a tight-knit community where sign language is central to communication. This community offers support, understanding, and a sense of belonging to individuals who share similar experiences of deafness. Sign language also serves as a bridge connecting deaf individuals, enabling them to participate in various social, educational, and professional settings.

1.3 Visual-Spatial language

The study of visual-spatial languages presents a fascinating inquiry into communication, transcending the boundaries between the auditory and vocal modalities. Although sign languages, frequently identified as the most prominent examples of this classification, barely touch upon the breadth of vision-spatial linguistic phenomena, they nevertheless serve as a valuable starting point for further investigation.

As shown in Fig. 1.2, visual-spatial languages utilize the visual and spatial dimensions for communication [18]. Unlike spoken languages, meaning is primarily constructed through auditory patterns, while visual-spatial languages rely on visual patterns, configurations, and movements in space [4]. These languages' semantics, grammar, and pragmatics are intricately tied to the spatial and visual modalities employed.

Although sign languages are the most prominent visual-spatial languages, they also encompass other systems that utilize visual cues for communication. For instance, indigenous tribes might use systematic patterns of drawings, totems, or body markings as media of communication that carry specific meanings and narratives [4].

The use of visual-spatial language has been found to influence cognitive processes. For instance, users often demonstrate heightened spatial cognition, visual memory, and even unique neural activation patterns compared with exclusive users of spoken language [19]. These cognitive variations underscore the profound ways in which our linguistic environments shape our minds. While rich and varied, visual-spatial languages present unique challenges, particularly in a world dominated by spoken and written communication. Preservation, documentation, and education have become crucial, especially for less-common systems that might be on the brink of extinction. Conversely, the rise of visual media in modern society has offered new platforms and opportunities for these languages to thrive and evolve [20].

Visual-spatial languages, in various forms, reflect human communication's incredible adaptability and diversity. Their existence reminds us that language, in essence, is about connection, whether through sound, sight, or space.

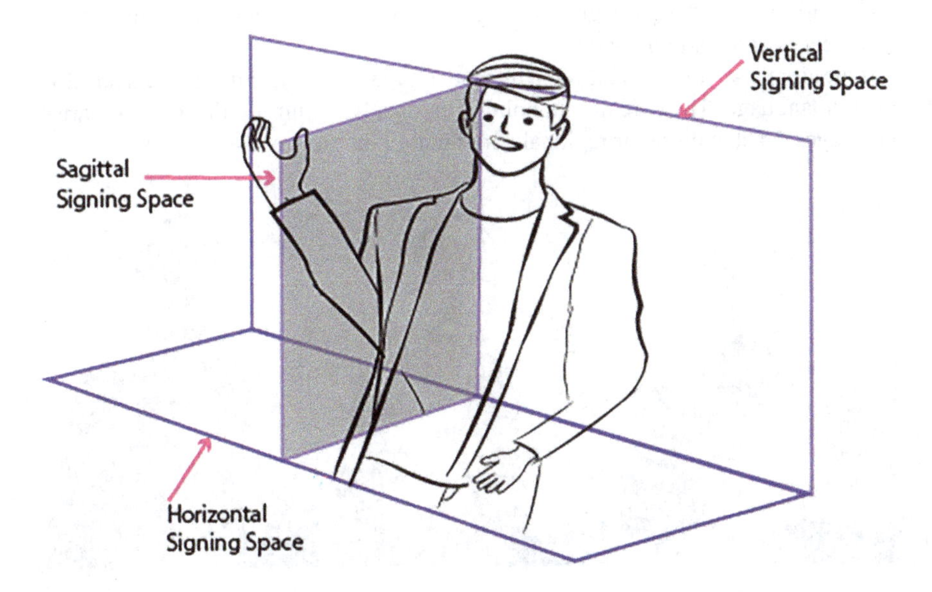

Fig. 1.2 Visual and space dimensions for communication

1.4 Defining Sign Languages

Sign language is a nonverbal communication method that relies on physical movement instead of spoken words. Visual-spatial language uses visible cues from the hands, eyes, facial expressions, and movements to convey meaning. Although sign language is primarily used by individuals who are deaf or hard of hearing, it is also used by many hearing people. Like spoken languages, sign languages have their own grammar and structural rules and have evolved. However, there is no universal sign language, and different countries have unique versions of sign languages specific to their regions and cultures. For instance, the ASL differs from Auslan in Australia and the BSL in the United Kingdom. A person fluent in ASL may need to understand a local version of sign language in Sydney, Australia, instead of different dialects or accents in spoken languages. More than 200 sign languages are spoken by more than 72 million deaf or hard-of-hearing individuals worldwide [21].

Figure 1.3 shows that the sign for "SCHOOL" in various sign languages exemplifies the diversity and uniqueness of gestural representations across cultures. In ASL, the sign is made by clapping the flat, open hands, together with a motion akin to clapping, a gesture reminiscent of a teacher calling for attention in the classroom. In contrast, BSL employs a fingered tap on the back of the other hand, symbolizing the raising of a hand in a school setting. Moving to Qatari Sign Language (QSL), the sign takes on a different form, incorporating a visual metaphor for the buildings or facilities associated with education. Meanwhile, French Sign Language (LSF) represents "*SCHOOL*" with a gesture that seems to capture the essence of academic life and learning, diverging from the other mentioned sign languages in form and conceptual underpinnings. Each variation of the sign for "SCHOOL" provides a window into how different sign language communities reflect their educational experiences and cultural contexts.

One significant distinction, often misunderstood by many, is the non-universality of sign language. They are not monolithic entities but comprise diverse and varied languages. Each cultural or regional community possesses a distinct sign language

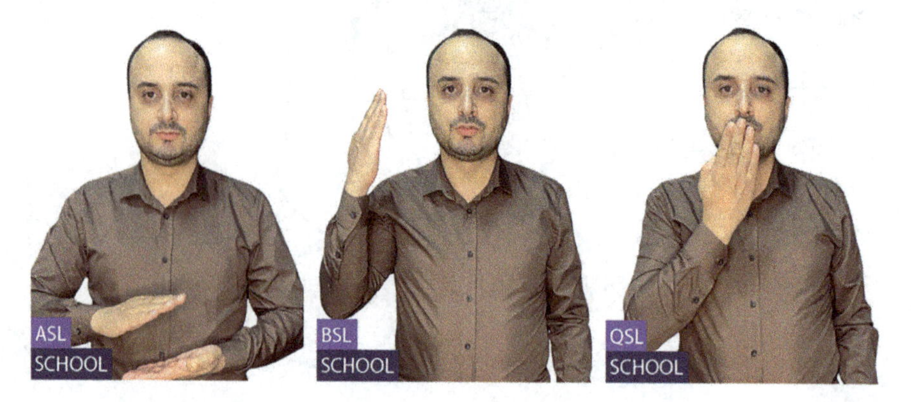

Fig. 1.3 The sign "SCHOOL" is a different sign languages. From left to right: ASL, BSL, QSL

rich in unique lexicons and grammatical structures, underscoring the diversity and depth of human linguistic expression [22].

Sign languages, distinct from the many communication methods employed by humans, exhibit expressions of complex linguistic systems rooted in visual-manual modality [23]. Rather than merely gestures, these languages are structured and intricate, evolving in response to cultural and societal influence. At the core of sign language lies manual articulation complemented by non-manual elements such as facial expressions and body posture [24]. This combination yields a rich communication tapestry in which each sign or gesture has a specific meaning organized by syntactic and morphological rules. As shown in Fig. 1.4, this well-defined structure distinguishes sign languages from simple gestural communication or mime, imbuing them with the complexity and depth characteristics of the spoken language [25].

Sign languages are distinct linguistic systems with evolutionary trajectories, as emphasized in [26]. They are not simply imitations or translations of spoken languages but autonomous systems with unique structures and properties. This was supported by Slobin [27], who argues that sign languages are problematic for the gestural origins theory of language evolution, as they exhibit the same complexities and evolutionary advantages as spoken languages. Carreiras adds to this by highlighting the typological differences between signed and spoken languages, with signed languages being head-marked and dependent on surrounding spoken/written

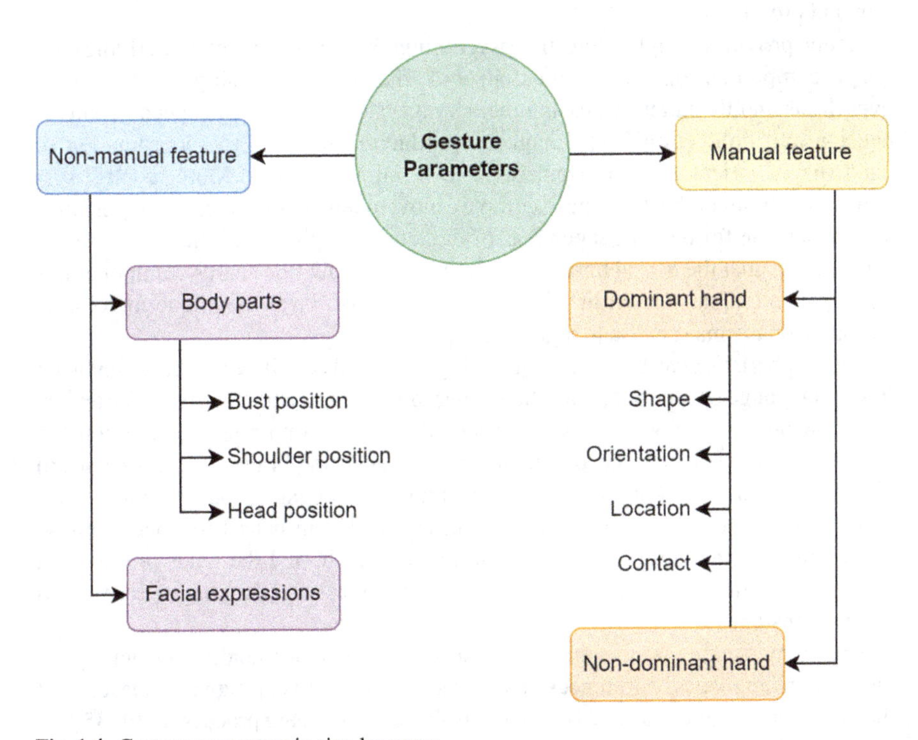

Fig. 1.4 Gesture parameters in sign language

languages [28]. Woll underscores the uniqueness of sign languages, noting that they have lexicons and grammar and are not derived from spoken languages [9].

It is crucial to underscore that sign languages are not merely imitations or translations of spoken language. Instead, they are autonomous linguistic systems with evolutionary trajectories that often diverge from the spoken languages of surrounding communities. This autonomy attests to human communication's infinite diversity, complexity, and flexibility. illustrates the various elements of a sign, which primarily consist of manual and non-manual components, thereby reflecting the distinctive signing conventions employed by different cultural communities.

1.5 Cognitive Processes in Sign Language Comprehension and Production

Understanding sign language requires advanced visual-spatial processing. The visual system must decipher gestural signals, including manual configurations, gestures, and facial expressions. Research on sign language comprehension and production has yielded several key findings. In [29, 30], the authors emphasized the importance of the age of acquisition and iconicity in sign language processing, with the latter also highlighting the role of the left hemisphere in sign language perception and production.

Izumi provides insights into the psycholinguistic mechanisms underlying language comprehension and production, with the former focusing on the output hypothesis and the latter discussing the neural systems involved in speech comprehension and production [31]. Language production involves the coordination of hand shapes, orientations, movements, and facial expressions. Motor control systems in the brain orchestrate these complex movements, with evidence suggesting a significant role for the language areas of the left hemisphere and the motor cortex. This implies that the neural basis of sign language production shares commonalities with spoken language regarding lateralization but also involves unique motor execution mechanisms specific to sign language.

José-Robertson et al. explore the neural systems and cognitive processes involved in sign language production, with the former identifying distinct systems for lexical selection and phonological encoding and the latter examining the relationship between comprehension and production processes in the brain [32]. Studies from [33, 34] further contribute to our understanding of language production and comprehension, with the former demonstrating an overlap in neural responses during the production and comprehension of narrative speech, and the latter proposing a model that links language production processes to language form and comprehension.

Emmorey's main findings include advancements in understanding the neurobiology of sign languages, differences in neural substrates between sign and speech, and the development of comprehensive models for sign language processing [4, 35].

Working memory plays a crucial role in the comprehension and production of sign language. Temporal and spatial aspects of signals must be retained in memory for processing and production. The complexity of sign language syntax and semantics modulates the cognitive load, necessitating efficient working memory systems. Neurocognitive studies have indicated that sign language users may develop enhanced spatial working memory capabilities, highlighting the mental benefits of bilingualism and bimodal language acquisition.

1.6 The Importance of Sign Languages

Beyond their linguistic uniqueness, sign languages occupy an essential position in society, acting as bridges of communication, cultural expression, and avenues for inclusion. Their significance, especially in deaf communities and cultures, cannot be overstated. For deaf and hard-of-hearing individuals, sign languages are more than just a communication medium; they are integral to their identities and cultures [36].

Through sign language, members of these communities express their feelings, share their narratives, and connect deeply with their heritage. These languages provide a sense of belonging, ensuring that individuals are not isolated due to their hearing status. Furthermore, sign language plays a pivotal role in cognitive and educational development. Research has shown that when deaf children are exposed to sign language early, they exhibit enhanced mental abilities, literacy skills, and academic performance comparable to hearing peers [37].

In a society that prioritizes inclusivity, sign language is a powerful tool to foster understanding and reduce barriers between the deaf and hearing communities [38]. Recognizing and promoting sign languages is a testament to acknowledging and validating societies' rich cultural and linguistic diversity.

Moreover, when sign languages are integrated into mainstream education, public services, and the media, they not only benefit deaf individuals but also contribute to creating more informed and empathetic communities. This integration can foster environments where deaf individuals can actively participate in public discourse, employment, and social activities without prejudice or limitations.

Promoting sign language education for hearing individuals can open avenues for richer interpersonal interactions, create professional opportunities for interpreting and teaching, and foster an environment of mutual respect and understanding [8]. The value of sign languages extends beyond their linguistic attributes. They are emblematic of inclusion, experience, and cultural richness, ensuring that deaf individuals are active and valued members of broader societal tapestry.

1.7 A Brief History of Sign Languages

The history of sign languages is deeply intertwined with the history of deaf communities worldwide. While many might consider sign languages a relatively recent development, their roots trace back several centuries, reflecting the resilience, adaptability, and cultural richness of deaf communities. Evidence suggests that rudimentary forms of sign language exist in ancient civilizations. From historical texts in ancient Greece to artwork from Renaissance Europe, depictions and descriptions indicate the presence of sign-based communication systems [39].

By the eighteenth century, distinct sign languages had begun to emerge, particularly in Europe. For example, in France, Charles-Michel de l'Épée founded the first public school for deaf students in the 1760s, significantly developing the modern French Sign Language [40]. From Europe, knowledge and teaching methodologies have spread to other parts of the world, influencing the establishment of sign languages in various regions.

One of the most remarkable aspects of sign language is its rich diversity. Just as spoken languages differ across countries and regions, sign languages also vary and are distinct. For instance, ASL and BSL are vastly different despite countries sharing English as their spoken language [41].

The reasons for this diversity are manifold. Local deaf communities have historically developed sign languages because of their unique experiences, cultural influences, and isolation from other deaf groups. Over time, these isolated communication systems have evolved into fully-fledged complex languages that reflect the cultural nuances of their respective communities [42].

Regional variation often exists among countries. Because spoken dialects can vary within a single country, they can also be sign language dialects. These differences might manifest as unique signs, variations in hand shapes, or even differing grammatical structures, reflecting the influence of local customs, history, and intergroup interactions. The history of sign languages shows the dynamism and adaptability of human communication. From their ancient origins to modern intricacies and variations, sign languages testify to the importance of community, cultural expression, and the universal human need to communicate and connect.

1.8 Diversity and Dialects in Sign Languages

Regional variation in sign languages is a complex phenomenon influenced by various social and linguistic factors. From the study [43], the authors highlight schools' role in shaping these variations. This influence may wane due to social and policy changes. In [44], researchers further emphasized the impact of social factors such as age, region of origin, language background, and linguistic factors such as phonological processes and grammaticalization [45]. Moreover, the study from [46] provides specific examples of this variation, with [45] identifying a range of linguistic and social factors that condition variation in American Sign Language and [46] noting a decrease in regional lexical variants in British Sign Language, particularly among younger signers. These studies underscore sign language variation's rich and dynamic nature, reflecting the influence of local customs, history, and intergroup interactions.

1.9 Universality of Sign Languages

The universality of sign languages encompasses the idea that underlying principles and structures are common across them despite the vast diversity and multitude of sign languages worldwide. This concept underscores languages' linguistic complexity and richness and highlights their integral roles in human communication and cognition.

Sign languages, such as spoken languages, are natural languages that evolve organically within communities. Their syntax, morphology, and semantics were developed to meet the communicative needs of the deaf and hard-of-hearing individuals. The universality of sign languages lies in their shared linguistic features, such as the use of spatial grammar, classifiers, and non-manual signals, which are found across different sign languages despite geographical and cultural differences.

1.10 Conclusion

The world of sign and visual-spatial languages offers a captivating journey toward the breadth and depth of human communication. As explored in this chapter, sign languages are not merely gestural systems but complex linguistic entities with rich histories that vary across countries and communities. Their significance, particularly for deaf and hard-of-hearing individuals, transcends communication and plays a pivotal role in societal inclusion, identity, and culture.

Furthermore, exploring visual-spatial languages broadens our understanding of modalities through which humans convey meaning. From intricate patterns in space to the utilization of visual cues, these languages remind us of the versatility and adaptability inherent in our communicative abilities.

As we move forward, it is essential to recognize and value the importance of these languages, both in their cultural contexts and in the broader spectrum of linguistic studies. They challenge our preconceptions, enrich our global tapestry of communication, and underscore our universal human desire to connect, share, and understand. Through this understanding, we can better appreciate the complexities and diversities of the languages surrounding us, setting the stage for deeper exploration in subsequent chapters.

Quiz Time

1. What primarily distinguishes sign languages from spoken languages?

(A) Use of vocal cords
(B) Use of visual-spatial modalities
(C) Use of auditory cues

2. Which language is mentioned as a visual-spatial language that assists those with hearing impairment?

(A) British Sign Language (BSL)
(B) Makaton
(C) French Sign Language (LSF)

3. What is not, a characteristic feature of sign languages?

(A) Having its grammar
(B) Universal across all regions
(C) Utilized predominantly by deaf communities

4. According to the document, what does American Sign Language (ASL) rely heavily on hand gestures?

(A) Facial expressions
(B) Spoken words
(C) Written forms

5. Which systems facilitate comprehension through physical signals?

(A) Cued Speech
(B) American Sign Language
(C) Pidgin Signed English

6. What aspect of sign language is emphasized as being deeply ingrained within the culture and identity of deaf communities?

(A) Linguistic complexity
(B) Cultural and identity indicators
(C) Syntax similarities with spoken languages

7. What types of languages are described as having a lower linguistic complexity than sign languages?

(A) Auditory languages
(B) Visual-spatial languages
(C) Written languages

8. Which sign language is noted for its unique development in deaf schools in France?

(A) British Sign Language (BSL)
(B) French Sign Language (LSF)
(C) American Sign Language (ASL)

9. What is a significant challenge in studying visual-spatial languages?

(A) Easy integration with spoken languages
(B) Low interest in academic studies
(C) Overcoming preconceived notions about language structure

10. What significantly affects deafness and hearing loss?

(A) There was no significant impact on daily communication
(B) It primarily affects the elderly
(C) It profoundly affects an individual's ability to communicate and engage socially

References

1. Zeshan, U., Palfreyman, N.: Sign language typology. In: Sign Language Typology. pp. 178–216. Cambridge University Press (2017).
2. Johnson, R.E., Liddell, S.K.: A segmental framework for representing signs phonetically. Sign Language Studies. 11, 408–463 (2011).
3. Lucas, C.: The sociolinguistics of sign languages. (2001).
4. Emmorey, K.: Language, cognition, and the brain: Insights from sign language research. Psychology Press (2001).
5. Padden, C.A., Humphries, T.L.: Deaf in America: Voices from a culture. Harvard University Press (1988).
6. Mistry, M., Barnes, D.: The use of Makaton for supporting talk, through play, for pupils who have English as an Additional Language (EAL) in the Foundation Stage. Education 3-13. 41, 603–616 (2013). https://doi.org/10.1080/03004279.2011.631560.
7. Nicholls, G.H., Mcgill, D.L.: Cued Speech and the Reception of Spoken Language. J Speech Lang Hear Res. 25, 262–269 (1982). https://doi.org/10.1044/jshr.2502.262.
8. Ladd, P.: Sign Language: Communities and Cultures. In: Brown, K. (ed.) Encyclopedia of Language & Linguistics (Second Edition). pp. 296–303. Elsevier, Oxford (2006). https://doi.org/10.1016/B0-08-044854-2/00225-X.
9. Woll, B.: Applied Linguistics from the Perspective of Sign Language and Deaf Studies. White Rose University Press. (2019). https://doi.org/10.22599/BAAL1.d.
10. Dotter, F.: Sign languages and their communities now and in the future. des Zentrums für Gebärdensprache und Hörbehindertenkommunikation Band 22. 93 (2013).
11. Tucci, D.L., Merson, M.H., Wilson, B.S.: A Summary of the Literature on Global Hearing Impairment: Current Status and Priorities for Action. Otology & Neurotology. 31, 31 (2010). https://doi.org/10.1097/MAO.0b013e3181c0eaec.
12. Souza, P.: Speech Perception and Hearing Aids. In: Popelka, G.R., Moore, B.C.J., Fay, R.R., and Popper, A.N. (eds.) Hearing Aids. pp. 151–180. Springer International Publishing, Cham (2016). https://doi.org/10.1007/978-3-319-33036-5_6.
13. Davis, A., McMahon, C.M., Pichora-Fuller, K.M., Russ, S., Lin, F., Olusanya, B.O., Chadha, S., Tremblay, K.L.: Aging and Hearing Health: The Life-course Approach. The Gerontologist. 56, S256–S267 (2016). https://doi.org/10.1093/geront/gnw033.
14. López-Torres Hidalgo, J., Gras, C.B., Lapeira, J.T., Verdejo, M.Á.L., del Campo del Campo, J.M., Rabadán, F.E.: Functional status of elderly people with hearing loss. Archives of Gerontology and Geriatrics. 49, 88–92 (2009). https://doi.org/10.1016/j.archger.2008.05.006.
15. Olusanya, B.O., Davis, A.C., Hoffman, H.J.: Hearing loss grades and the International classification of functioning, disability and health. Bull World Health Organ. 97, 725–728 (2019). https://doi.org/10.2471/BLT.19.230367.

16. Wilson, B.S., Tucci, D.L., Merson, M.H., O'Donoghue, G.M.: Global hearing health care: new findings and perspectives. The Lancet. 390, 2503–2515 (2017). https://doi.org/10.1016/S0140-6736(17)31073-5.
17. Deafness And Hearing Loss Statistics, https://www.forbes.com/health/hearing-aids/deafness-statistics/, last accessed 2024/01/07.
18. Language, Cognition, and Deafness, https://www.routledge.com/Language-Cognition-and-Deafness/Rodda-Grove/p/book/9780898598773, last accessed 2024/04/07.
19. Newman, A.J., Bavelier, D., Corina, D., Jezzard, P., Neville, H.J.: A critical period for right hemisphere recruitment in American Sign Language processing. Nat Neurosci. 5, 76–80 (2002). https://doi.org/10.1038/nn775.
20. Meier, R.P., Cormier, K., Quinto-Pozos, D. eds: Modality and Structure in Signed and Spoken Languages. Cambridge University Press, Cambridge (2002). https://doi.org/10.1017/CBO9780511486777.
21. Farooq, U., Rahim, M.S.M., Sabir, N., Hussain, A., Abid, A.: Advances in machine translation for sign language: approaches, limitations, and challenges. Neural Comput & Applic. 33, 14357–14399 (2021). https://doi.org/10.1007/s00521-021-06079-3.
22. Anderson, S.: Languages: A Very Short Introduction. Oxford University Press (2012). https://doi.org/10.1093/actrade/9780199590599.001.0001.
23. Perniss, P., Özyürek, A., Morgan, G.: The Influence of the Visual Modality on Language Structure and Conventionalization: Insights From Sign Language and Gesture. Topics in Cognitive Science. 7, 2–11 (2015). https://doi.org/10.1111/tops.12127.
24. Sandler, W.: The Phonological Organization of Sign Languages. Language and Linguistics Compass. 6, 162–182 (2012). https://doi.org/10.1002/lnc3.326.
25. Morgan, G.: On language acquisition in speech and sign: development of combinatorial structure in both modalities. Frontiers in Psychology. 5, (2014).
26. Sandler, W.: The uniformity and diversity of language: Evidence from sign language. Lingua. 120, 2727–2732 (2010). https://doi.org/10.1016/j.lingua.2010.03.015.
27. Emmorey, K.: Sign languages are problematic for a gestural origins theory of language evolution. Behavioral and Brain Sciences. 28, 130–131 (2005). https://doi.org/10.1017/S0140525X05270036.
28. Slobin, D.I.: Breaking the Molds: Signed Languages and the Nature of Human Language. Sign Language Studies. 8, 114–130 (2008).
29. Carreiras, M.: Sign Language Processing. Language and Linguistics Compass. 4, 430–444 (2010). https://doi.org/10.1111/j.1749-818X.2010.00192.x.
30. Rönnberg, J., Söderfeldt, B., Risberg, J.: The cognitive neuroscience of signed language. Acta Psychologica. 105, 237–254 (2000). https://doi.org/10.1016/S0001-6918(00)00063-9.
31. Izumi, S.: Comprehension and Production Processes in Second Language Learning: In Search of the Psycholinguistic Rationale of the Output Hypothesis. Applied Linguistics. 24, 168–196 (2003). https://doi.org/10.1093/applin/24.2.168.
32. San José-Robertson, L., Corina, D.P., Ackerman, D., Guillemin, A., Braun, A.R.: Neural systems for sign language production: Mechanisms supporting lexical selection, phonological encoding, and articulation. Human Brain Mapping. 23, 156–167 (2004). https://doi.org/10.1002/hbm.20054.
33. Silbert, L.J., Honey, C.J., Simony, E., Poeppel, D., Hasson, U.: Coupled neural systems underlie the production and comprehension of naturalistic narrative speech. Proceedings of the National Academy of Sciences. 111, E4687–E4696 (2014). https://doi.org/10.1073/pnas.1323812111.
34. MacDonald, M.C.: How language production shapes language form and comprehension. Front. Psychol. 4, (2013). https://doi.org/10.3389/fpsyg.2013.00226.
35. Emmorey, K.: New Perspectives on the Neurobiology of Sign Languages. Front. Commun. 6, (2021). https://doi.org/10.3389/fcomm.2021.748430.
36. Padden, C., Humphries, T.: Inside Deaf Culture. Harvard University Press (2005). https://doi.org/10.2307/j.ctvjz83v3.

37. Mayberry, R.I., Lock, E.: Age constraints on first versus second language acquisition: evidence for linguistic plasticity and epigenesis. Brain Lang. 87, 369–384 (2003). https://doi.org/10.1016/s0093-934x(03)00137-8.
38. Solomon, A., Skuttnab-Kangas, T.: Deaf Gain: Raising the Stakes for Human Diversity. University of Minnesota Press (2014).
39. Plann, S.: A Silent Minority: Deaf Education in Spain, 1550-1835. University of California Press, Berkeley (1997).
40. Lane, H.: When the Mind Hears: A History of the Deaf. Vintage, New York (1989).
41. Kyle, J.G., Woll, B., Pullen, G., Maddix, F.: Sign Language: The Study of Deaf People and their Language. Cambridge University Press, Cambridge (1988).
42. Lucas, C., Valli, C.: 2 - Language Contact in the American Deaf Community. In: Lucas, C. (ed.) The Sociolinguistics of the Deaf Community. pp. 11–40. Academic Press, San Diego (1989). https://doi.org/10.1016/B978-0-12-458045-9.50008-2.
43. Eichmann, H., Rosenstock, R.: Regional Variation in German Sign Language: The Role of Schools (Re-)Visited. Sign Language Studies. 14, 175–202 (2014).
44. Schembri, A., Johnston, T.: Sociolinguistic Variation and Change in Sign Languages. In: Bayley, R., Cameron, R., and Lucas, C. (eds.) The Oxford Handbook of Sociolinguistics. p. 0. Oxford University Press (2013). https://doi.org/10.1093/oxfordhb/9780199744084.013.0025.
45. Bayley, R., Lucas, C., Rose, M.: Phonological variation in American Sign Language: The case of 1 handshape. Language Variation and Change. 14, 19–53 (2002). https://doi.org/10.1017/S0954394502141020.
46. Stamp, R., Schembri, A., Fenlon, J., Rentelis, R., Woll, B., Cormier, K.: Lexical Variation and Change in British Sign Language. PLOS ONE. 9, e94053 (2014). https://doi.org/10.1371/journal.pone.0094053.

Chapter 2
Structure of Sign Language

2.1 Introduction

While visually captivating and gesturally expressive, sign languages are underpinned by a profoundly intricate linguistic structure, echoing the complexities of spoken language. A dive beneath the surface of gestures and signs unveils a world with rules, patterns, and meanings, all working harmoniously to facilitate robust communication within and beyond the deaf community.

This chapter presents the structural framework of sign language concisely. The objective is to provide a fundamental understanding of their internal structures by systematically examining their constituent parts, from the foundational units of signs to the sociocultural contexts in which they are utilized. As this exploration commences, we will explore phonology and uncover the essential components that make up these signs. We then proceed to morphology and syntax, illuminating how signs are formed and combined to create coherent, meaningful sentences.

Our journey extends beyond fundamental structures to encompass semantics, wherein the intrinsic nature of each sign is elucidated, and the interplay between signs engenders comprehensive narratives. Moreover, as language serves not only as an instrument for disseminating information but also as a medium for social interaction, our investigation culminates in the examination of pragmatics, revealing the multifaceted manner in which sign languages adapt, evolve, and resonate within diverse communicative contexts.

This chapter explores the intricacies of sign language structure, providing a comprehensive understanding of the richness and complexity that sign languages embody. This knowledge will serve as a crucial foundation, paving the way for further exploration of sign language in subsequent chapters.

A. Othman, *Sign Language Processing*,
https://doi.org/10.1007/978-3-031-68763-1_2

2.2 Phonology

At the heart of all languages, spoken or signed, lies the study of phonology. This discipline investigates the systematic arrangement of sounds in spoken languages and the corresponding organization of meaningful units in sign languages. In the case of sign languages, these units are not acoustic but instead composed of distinct hand shapes, locations, movements, and facial expressions. These elements work harmoniously to serve as essential structures for the sign-language framework.

A comparison of spoken and signed languages has revealed both modality-independent linguistic and modality-dependent structures [1]. In Dutch Sign Language (in Dutch: Nederlandse Gebarentaal or NGT), phonological analysis has proposed a model with fewer phonological distinctions, achieved through phonetic implementation rules and semantic pre-specification [2]. A sonority cycle in American Sign Language has been identified, with phonological elements categorized based on hand shape, location, and movement [1]. The interface between morphology and phonology in signed languages has been explored, highlighting the role of phonological constraints in morphological processes [3]. Due to their non-distinctive properties and iconicity, the need for a smaller set of phonological features in sign languages has been emphasized [4].

Figure 2.1 illustrates the execution of the sign for "CAN", which is demonstrated across various channels, as detailed later. This multifaceted approach to signing "CAN" encompasses a range of modalities, each contributing to overall comprehension and conveyance of the sign. These channels, which include handshape, movement, orientation, location, and facial expressions, work in unison to provide a comprehensive representation of the sign "CAN," highlighting the intricacies involved in its execution:

- **Handshape**: This refers to the specific shape of the hands when producing a sign. Different hand shapes can change the meaning of a sign, as different vowels or consonants can change the meaning of a word in spoken language.
- **Orientation**: This involves the direction the palms or fingers face during the sign. The orientation can be towards or away from the signer, up, down, or to the side, and like a hand shape, it can significantly alter the meaning of a sign.

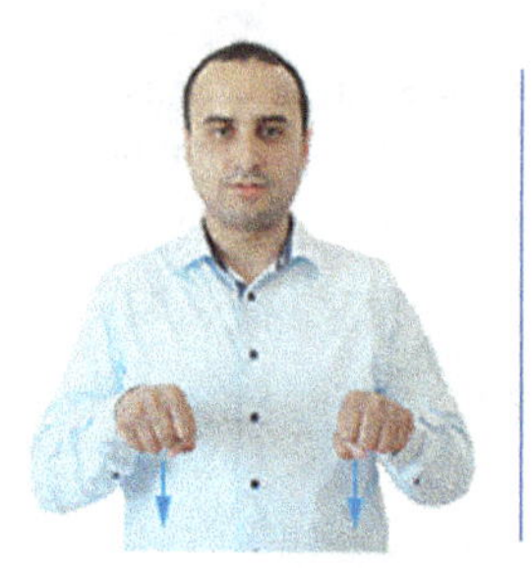

- Configuration: Closed fists
- Location: In front of the torso, near the chest or shoulders
- Orientation: Knuckles facing outwards
- Movement: Simple, downward movement of both fists
- Facial Expression: Affirmative

Fig. 2.1 The sign "CAN" in ASL

- **Location**: This refers to the location in the signing space where a sign is produced, such as in front of the face, on the body, or in the neutral space in front of the signer. Location helps differentiate signs that might otherwise be similar in hand shape, orientation, and movement.
- **Movement**: Sign languages use various movements, including direction, path, and manner (smooth, fast, or slow). Movement is crucial for expressing different concepts and can change the tense or aspects of verbs, among other things.
- **Facial Expressions**: In sign languages, facial expressions are not just emotional indicators but are integral to grammar and lexicon, conveying distinctions in meaning, mood, tense, and sentence type (e.g., declarative, interrogative).

Understanding the phonology of sign languages is similar to acquiring the alphabet of a spoken language. The distinct characteristics of these elemental units lay the foundation for forming more complex structures and meanings. As we delve deeper into the intricacies of sign language, appreciating these fundamental building blocks will prove instrumental in grasping more advanced aspects of morphology, syntax, semantics, and pragmatics.

2.3 Morphology

Morphology in sign language refers to the study of the internal structure of signs and how they can be analyzed into their most minor meaningful units, known as morphemes. Like spoken languages, sign languages exhibit morphological processes, such as derivation and inflection, enabling new signs to form or modify existing signs to convey different grammatical categories. Derivational morphology in sign language can involve hand shape, movement, or location changes to create new words from existing ones. In contrast, inflectional morphology often involves modifications to indicate tense, number, aspect, or other grammatical features. These morphological processes demonstrate sign languages' linguistic richness and complexity, highlighting their status as fully-fledged natural languages with unique grammatical systems.

In the literature, [5, 6] highlighted the use of simultaneous morphemes, which are particularly rich in sign languages. This was further explored in [7], who emphasized the role of physical properties in sign language typology. [6] also discusses sequential and simultaneous morphological structures in sign languages, with the former being more derivational and the latter being more inflectional. This is supported by [8], who identified two types of non-concatenative morphology in signed languages. [9] extended this discussion by applying a construction morphology approach to sign language analysis, which provides a uniform analysis of the core and classifier signs.

Morphemes in Sign Language

Morphemes in sign language constitute the most minor units, pivotal in signs' linguistic structure and formation. These morphemes can be manual, involving hand shapes, movements, locations, and orientations, or non-manual, involving facial expressions and body postures. Sign languages use these morphemes in free and bound forms to construct a wide array of meaningful expressions. Free morphemes can stand alone as independent signs analogous to words in spoken languages. In contrast, bound morphemes attach to other signs to modify their meaning or grammatical function, similar to the prefixes or suffixes in spoken languages. This dual structure of morphemes in sign language underscores its complexity and flexibility, allowing nuanced and precise communication.

When altering the meaning of a sign by changing its movement, modification of the movement itself constitutes a morpheme. This morpheme was classified as a process morpheme. The sign "CHAIR"[1] is composed of two morphemes: the free morpheme "SIT"[2] and the process morpheme "double movement."

Fingerspelling

Fingerspelling involves using hand movements to represent letters of the alphabet, allowing for the spelling of words for which there are no established signs, including proper nouns, technical terms, and new or foreign words, thus serving as a critical bridge between sign language and the written form of spoken language. Figure 2.2 displays the sign language alphabet, showcasing the unique hand shapes used to represent each letter as an example of ASL [10]. By combining individual signs for letters, signers can convey an extensive range of vocabulary, ensuring clarity and precision in communication. This technique is integral to sign language and enhances its expressiveness and versatility.

An example of fingerspelling using gloss notation (the notation will be explained in Chap. 4: Sign Language Processing Part 1) can be demonstrated with the word "CAT." In gloss notation, fingerspelling is typically indicated by listing each letter of the word spelled out, often separated by hyphens or spaced out, and enclosed in square brackets to differentiate it from regular signs. Thus, the fingerspelling of "CAT" would be represented in gloss notation as: [C-A-T]. This indicates that the signer sequentially forms handshapes for letters C, A, and T to spell out the word "CAT" using sign language fingerspelling.

[1] The sign "CHAIR": https://babysignlanguage.com/dictionary/chair/

[2] The sign "SIT": https://babysignlanguage.com/dictionary/sit/

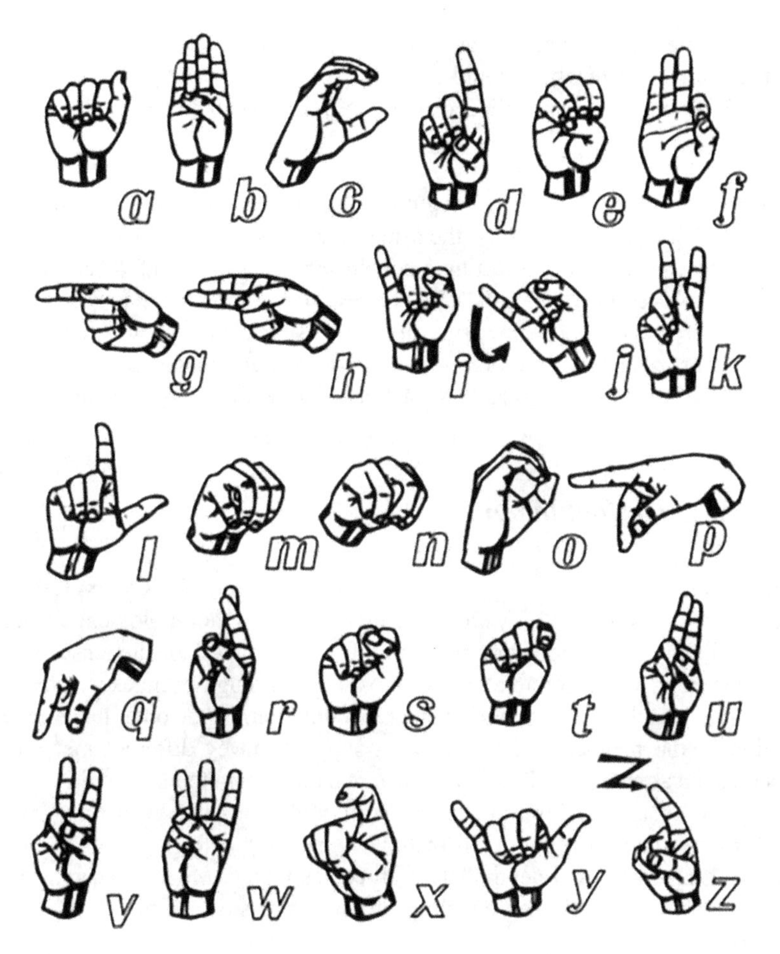

Fig. 2.2 Fingerspelling in American Sign Language (Coloringbuddymike, CC BY-SA 3.0 <https://creativecommons.org/licenses/by-sa/3.0>, via Wikimedia Commons)

Compound Signs

Compound signs in sign languages combine two or more existing signs to create a new sign with a distinct meaning. This morphological process mirrors compounding in spoken languages, in which two words merge to produce a new word. In sign language, compounding involves integrating elements such as hand shapes, movements, and locations from the original signs. The resulting compound sign often undergoes phonological reduction, meaning that certain features of the original sign may be simplified or omitted in the compound form. This linguistic mechanism expands the lexicon of sign languages, allowing for efficient and creative expression of complex concepts through a single manual gesture. Thus, compound signs play a crucial role in the evolution and dynamism of sign-language vocabulary.

An example of a compound sign in sign language as illustrated in Fig. 2.3, represented using gloss notation, could be the compound sign for "WEEKEND." This sign combines the signs for "WEEK" and "END." This can be represented as

WEEK + END = WEEKEND.

In this compound sign, "WEEK" might be signed with a specific hand shape and movement that denotes 7 days. At the same time, "END" could involve a different hand shape or movement, indicating a conclusion or termination. When these two signs are combined into "WEEKEND," the resulting compound may simplify each element to create a new, distinct sign that effectively communicates the weekend concept. This example illustrates how compound signs merge the phonological aspects of their constituent signs to form a new sign with a unique meaning.

Inflection and Modulation

Inflection and modulation in sign language involve altering signs to express grammatical relationships or modify words' meaning, akin to morphological changes in spoken language. Inflection pertains to modifying a sign to indicate tense, number, aspect, mood, or other grammatical features, often through changes in movement, orientation, or adding specific morphemes. Modulation, on the other hand, refers to variation in the manner or intensity of a sign to convey different meanings or nuances, such as changing the speed or size of a movement to indicate the degree of an adjective or adverb. Both inflection and modulation are critical for conveying complex information and subtle distinctions in meaning, allowing users to communicate with precision and depth. These processes underscore sign languages' linguistic richness and flexibility, enabling various expressions within a visual-spatial modality.

Research on inflection in sign language has revealed that it is processed componentially, similar to spoken language [11]. The use of inflectional morphemes in manual English by hearing-impaired children is influenced by the mothers' use of these morphemes [12]. Sign languages, including the American Sign Language, exhibit simultaneous and sequential morphological structures, with the former

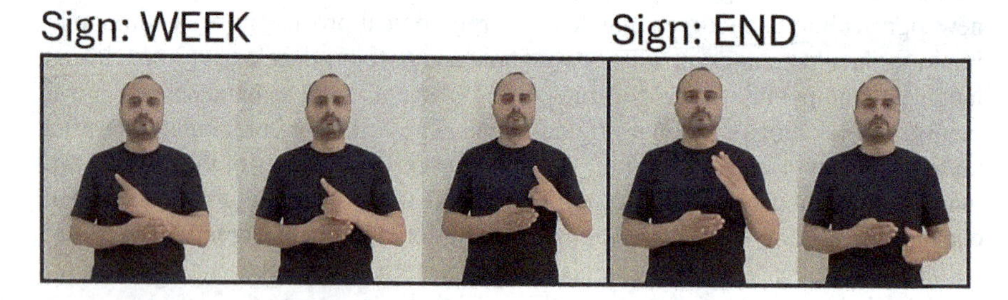

Fig. 2.3 Compound sign "WEEKEND" in American Sign Language

being largely inflectional [5]. ASL also exploits morphological possibilities, such as compounding and reduplication, and uses ion morphs to create related signs [13].

Modulation of sign language has revealed several key findings. In [14], the influence of the visual modality on language structure and conventionalization was investigated, with signers being more sensitive to hand shape and movement. Corina further supports this [15], finding that sign language production activates brain regions similar to spoken language, indicating stable left-hemisphere activation regardless of articulatory demands.

An example of inflection and modulation in sign language illustrates how a verb is modified to convey tense, aspect, or plurality. Consider the verb "to run," which might be glossed simply as RUN in its base form. To inflect this verb to express the concept of "running repeatedly" or "run habitually," an aspectual inflection can be added. RUN++ can represent this. The "++" indicates a modification of the base sign through repeated movement, suggesting a habitual or ongoing action. This inflection signals that the running action is not a one-time event but occurs regularly or continuously over time.

Another example of inflection and modulation in sign language is the concept of size. Consider the adjective "BIG." In its standard form, it may be glossed as BIG. To modulate this sign to express "extremely big" or "gigantic," the sign can be altered by significantly increasing the movement or the spatial extent of the sign. This can be represented in the gloss notation as BIG+++. Here, "+++" signifies substantial modulation from the base sign, indicating a larger size or extent. By expanding the physical space used in the sign or the dynamic of the movement, the signer effectively communicates a degree of size well beyond the ordinary meaning of "big."

This technique of inflection and modulation allows signers to convey nuances and variations in meaning purely through visual-manual modality, demonstrating the expressive capacity of sign language.

Derivational Processes

Derivational processes in sign language refer to morphological operations that create new words from existing ones, expanding the lexicon and allowing for linguistic creativity and precision. These processes included affixation, compounding, and reduplication. Affixation involves the addition of prefixes or suffixes to a base sign, altering its meaning, or creating a word in a new grammatical category. Compounding combines two or more signs into a new sign, often with a meaning related to but distinct from its components. Reduplication modifies a sign through the repetition or variation of its movement or other features, denoting pluralization, intensity, or aspectual changes. Through these derivational mechanisms, sign languages generate a rich array of vocabulary items expressing complex concepts, actions, and attributes, demonstrating a language's dynamism and adaptability to communicative needs.

An example of a derivational process in sign language is converting a verb to an adjective. Consider the verb "MOVE." To derive an adjective meaning "movable," a derivational morpheme that indicates the quality or characteristic can be appended. This process can be represented in GLOSS notation as MOVE-ABLE.

The suffix "-ABLE" attached to the base verb "MOVE" transforms it into an adjective, resulting in "movable." This example demonstrates the use of derivational morphology to modify the meaning of a sign by denoting an action to describe a quality or capability related to that action.

Classifiers

Classifiers (CL) in sign language are a group of hand shapes used to represent general categories of objects, people, places, or concepts, as well as their orientation, movement, and relationship to one another within the spatial context of the signer's narrative. These handshapes are not standalone signs but are employed within the structure of signed sentences to provide descriptive or locative information that complements the narrative. There are several classifiers, including object classifiers, which denote objects or people; locative classifiers, which describe a location or the distribution of items in space; and movement classifiers, which illustrate how an object moves or moves in space. In addition, body classifiers represent parts of the body or whole-body movements. Classifiers allow signers to convey complex visual-spatial information efficiently and vividly, making them essential to sign language's grammatical structure and expressive power.

An example of a classifier in sign language involves describing a moving car as the following scenario:

- Establish the object: CAR (using the specific sign for "CAR").
- Introduce the classifier: CL:3 ("3" handshape classifier to represent vehicles).
- Describe the movement: CL:3 moves forward.

The notation "CL:3 moves forward" uses the "3" handshape (with the thumb, index, and middle finger extended, resembling the shape of a vehicle) as a classifier to depict the car's motion. This classifier handshape is then moved through the signer's visual space to indicate that the car is moving forward. Using a classifier visually represents the car's action, enhancing the narrative's descriptive detail and spatial orientation.

There are several primary categories of classifiers, each with a distinct function:

- Object Classifiers: represent objects or people with various shapes and sizes. For example, a flat hand may represent a flat surface or vehicle, whereas an upright index finger can denote a person standing.
- Locative Classifiers: describe the location of objects or the spatial relationships between them. They can indicate where something is situated or how items are arranged relative to each other.

- Plural Classifiers: used to depict groups of objects or people and their distribution in space. These classifiers can show the arrangement of objects, such as items lined up in a row or randomly scattered.
- Element Classifiers: convey information about natural elements or substances such as water, fire, smoke, and wind, illustrating the movement or texture of these elements.
- Body Classifiers: represent parts of the body or whole-body actions. They can show how a body part moves or is positioned in space.
- Movement Classifiers: illustrate how an object or person moves within a space, including the direction, manner, and speed of movement.
- Instrument Classifiers: show how an object is manipulated or used, often indicating the type of grip or action performed with tools or utensils.
- Size and Shape Specifiers: provide specific details about the size, shape, or orientation of objects, enhancing descriptive accuracy and visual clarity in narratives.

Many studies have explored using classifiers in sign languages, revealing their complex and rule-governed nature [16]. [17] investigates into the discrete, rule-governed nature of classifier systems, with the latter questioning the treatment of these aspects as discrete morphemes. [18] provides insights into the psycholinguistic mechanisms of classifier processing and the similarities in morphology and constructions across sign languages. Cogill-Koez presents a model of classifier predicates as visual representation [19], while Koenders discusses using verbal, noun, and numeral classifiers in Hong Kong Sign Language [20].

2.4 Syntax

Syntax in sign language encompasses the rules and principles that govern the structure of sentences, dictating the arrangement of words and phrases to convey complex ideas coherently and cohesively. Unlike spoken languages, which rely primarily on linear sequencing of sounds, sign languages exploit their modality's spatial and visual nature to encode syntactic information. This includes using three-dimensional space to establish referents for subjects, objects, and locations and manipulating sign order, facial expressions, and body posture to indicate grammatical relationships and sentence types.

For instance, the topic-comment structure is prevalent, where the topic is introduced before its commentary or predicate, often supported by non-manual markers. Additionally, sign languages employ classifiers within their syntax to provide detailed descriptions of actions, locations, and the characteristics of subjects and objects within a narrative. The flexibility in sign order, influenced by context and emphasis, showcases the dynamic nature of sign language syntax, which, while distinct from spoken language syntax, adheres to universal linguistic principles, ensuring clarity, efficiency, and expressiveness in communication. Through these syntactic mechanisms, sign languages construct richly detailed and nuanced expressions, reflecting their users' cognitive and creative capabilities.

Linear and Nonlinear Structure

The distinction between linear and nonlinear structures within sign languages embodies a fundamental aspect of their linguistic architecture, exploiting the visual-spatial modality to enhance communicative depth and efficiency. Linear structure pertains to the sequential arrangement of signs, where the order of elements is critical to meaning and grammatical integrity, much like the syntactic ordering in spoken languages. However, the essence of sign languages also lies in their capacity for nonlinear structuring, which breaks away from mere sequentially to embrace spatial organization and the simultaneous conveyance of multiple pieces of information. This nonlinear approach leverages the signer's visual field and body as a canvas, where spatial locations can represent different entities or concepts, and movements between these points can depict relationships or actions, all within a single gestural expression. Simultaneity in sign languages is not just a feature but a necessity, allowing for the layering of meanings through classifiers, directional verbs, and non-manual signals such as facial expressions and body orientation, which, together, can articulate complex scenarios or nuanced states of being in a compact and integrated manner.

For instance, consider the construction of a sentence that describes someone giving a book to a friend, represented in gloss notation as: ME GIVE-TO[arc] YOU BOOK.

Here, "ME" and "YOU" establish the participants linearly, while "GIVE-TO[arc]" employs a directional verb to indicate the action and its direction—nonlinearly—from the signer to the recipient, integrated with the object "BOOK." The arc movement of the verb encapsulates the action's trajectory, blending the linear progression of the narrative with the spatial dynamics of the verb's directionality. This example underlines how sign languages meld linear and nonlinear structures, harnessing their unique modality to efficiently convey rich, multidimensional messages.

Spatial Grammar

Spatial grammar in sign languages capitalizes on using physical space to organize and convey linguistic information, embodying a distinctive feature that sets these languages apart from their spoken counterparts. This spatial organization encompasses several dimensions, including the establishment of locations to represent referents (persons, places, things), the use of movement between these locations to indicate actions or relationships, and the deployment of spatial configurations to express grammatical functions such as verb tense, aspect, or sentence structure. Through spatial grammar, sign languages achieve a high degree of expressivity and specificity, allowing signers to create vivid, visually oriented narratives that can convey complex spatial relationships and sequences of events with clarity and precision. The manipulation of space is not merely illustrative but is grammatically integral, encoding subject-object-verb relationships, plural forms, temporal sequences, and more within the spatial arrangement of signs. This use of space as a grammatical tool reflects the inherently visual-spatial nature of sign languages, providing a rich linguistic resource for conveying detailed information and nuanced meaning.

An illustrative example might involve describing two people meeting and conversing in a park as follows:

TWO-PERSON MEET PARK IX-LEFT PERSON-A IX-RIGHT PERSON-B CONVERSE.

In this sequence, "TWO-PERSON MEET PARK" sets the scene linearly, while "IX-LEFT" and "IX-RIGHT" establish spatial points for "PERSON-A" and "PERSON-B," respectively. The verb "CONVERSE" then utilizes these spatial referents to indicate the interaction between the two individuals. It employs spatial grammar to depict who is involved in the conversation and where they are positioned relative to each other. This example demonstrates how spatial grammar in sign language conveys action and location and integrates grammatical structure and relational dynamics within the spatial modality.

Role Shifting

Role shifting in sign language is a sophisticated narrative device that allows signers to assume the perspectives and personas of different characters within a story, facilitating a dynamic and immersive storytelling experience. This technique involves the physical and linguistic adaptation of the signer to represent different characters' viewpoints, emotions, and actions, effectively creating a visual and spatial dialogue or interaction among multiple characters without the need for verbal narration. Role shifting is achieved through changes in body orientation, facial expressions, and the spatial positioning of signs to delineate one character from another. This method enriches narrative complexity and enhances the clarity of interactions and emotional nuances between characters, providing a clear visual distinction of narrative roles within a single spatial frame. The strategic use of space, coupled with non-manual signals and directional verbs, enables signers to convey subtle shifts in narrative perspective, making role shifting a key component of sign language grammar that underscores its capacity for nuanced and multifaceted communication.

An example in gloss notation to illustrate role shifting could involve a conversation between two people, person A, and person B, about going to a movie, as follows:

PERSON-A IX-me WANT GO MOVIE, IX-you?

Shift body orientation to assume PERSON-B's role:

PERSON-B IX-me YES, IX-you WANT WHAT-TIME GO?

Here, "PERSON-A" and "PERSON-B" are identified initially with index pointing (IX-me for self-reference and IX-you for addressing the other). The narrative shifts between these two by changing the signer's body orientation and gaze to reflect the speaker's perspective at each point in the dialogue. Using "IX-me" and "IX-you" within each role shift helps clarify the speaker and addressee, thereby maintaining the dialogue's coherence. This example demonstrates how role shifting in sign language enables a clear and engaging portrayal of conversational exchanges and character dynamics.

Negation

Negation in sign language employs specific manual and non-manual markers to convey the negation of statements, questions, or commands, thereby expressing concepts of non-existence, prohibition, or contradiction. These markers include specific signs for negation, such as NOT or NONE, head shakes, and facial expressions that collectively modify the meaning of sentences to indicate negation. The integration of these elements is crucial for clear communication, as the placement and timing of negation markers can alter the scope and focus of negation within the sentence. This multi-modal approach to negation allows signers to express nuances of meaning, including the degree of negation or emphasis, through visual gestures and facial expressions. The flexibility in the expression of negation in sign languages showcases their complexity and depth, enabling signers to convey detailed and nuanced perspectives and reactions.

An example of negation in ASL might be:

ME WANT GO MOVIE, IX-you? HEAD-SHAKE.

In this sentence, "ME WANT GO MOVIE" is made as a proposition about wanting to go to the movie. The addition of "IX-you?" invites a response, and the subsequent "HEAD-SHAKE" functions as a non-manual negation marker, indicating a negative response or refusal. The head shake, in conjunction with the questioning expression, effectively negates the proposition or inquiry, signaling disagreement or the unwillingness of the second person to participate. This example illustrates how sign language utilizes both manual signs and non-manual signals to articulate complex linguistic functions like negation, enhancing the expressive capability of the language.

Question

Question formation in sign language incorporates various linguistic tools to differentiate interrogative sentences from declarative or imperative ones. This distinction is achieved through specific syntactic structures, manual signs for question words (wh-questions), and non-manual markers such as raised eyebrows, forward leans, or eye gaze, which are integral to signaling the interrogative nature of a sentence. The positioning of question words often occurs at the beginning or end of sentences, depending on the type of question being asked. Yes/no questions rely heavily on non-manual signals, whereas wh-questions utilize specific signs for who, what, where, when, why, and how at the sentence's start or end. This system allows signers to delineate questions from statements, facilitating precise and effective communication. The strategic use of space and classifier elements can further clarify the subject matter of questions, making questions in sign language an affluent area of linguistic structure and expression. An example of a question in ASL can be:

YOUR NAME WHAT? (Eyebrows up)

In this example, the question "WHAT" is used to inquire about the name of the person being addressed, with the non-manual marker of raised eyebrows throughout the sign indicating that a question is being asked. The syntax "YOUR NAME WHAT" with the non-manual signal marks this sentence as a wh-question, explicitly asking for information about the person's name. This example demonstrates how sign languages utilize manual and non-manual components to form questions, allowing for nuanced and effective communication.

Complex Sentences

Complex sentences in sign language, like spoken ones, combine multiple clauses to convey relationships of cause, condition, time, and contrast among ideas. These sentences may incorporate coordinating and subordinating conjunctions, relative clauses, and conditionals, facilitating the expression of nuanced and multifaceted ideas within a single utterance. The spatial and visual nature of sign languages allows for unique mechanisms to denote these complex relationships, such as through the use of space to establish temporal or causal sequences, classifier constructions to represent actions and actors across clauses, and non-manual signals like facial expressions and body posture to indicate conditional or hypothetical scenarios. Forming complex sentences in sign language exemplifies the language's capacity for depth and precision in communication, enabling signers to articulate detailed narratives, sophisticated arguments, and intricate descriptions. The modality of sign language, with its spatial grammar and visual immediacy, enriches the conveyance of complex ideas, making it a robust and expressive means of human communication.

An example of a complex sentence in ASL could be structured as follows:

IF IX-me FINISH WORK, IX-me GO MOVIE.

In this sentence, the conditional "IF" introduces the first clause, establishing a condition with "IX-me FINISH WORK," which is then followed by the consequence "IX-me GO MOVIE." Using index pointing (IX-me) clarifies the subject across both clauses, while spatial orientation and non-manual signals like facial expressions could further indicate the conditional nature of the statement. This example showcases how complex sentence structures in sign language enable signers to convey conditional relationships and hypothetical situations effectively.

Clause Combining

Clause combining in sign language entails the syntactic process of joining two or more clauses to form complex syntactic constructions, facilitating the expression of elaborate and interconnected ideas. This linguistic mechanism allows signers to articulate relationships between events, actions, and states within a coherent narrative framework, such as causality, temporality, conditionality, and contrast. Sign languages employ a variety of means for clause combining, including conjunctions, non-manual markers such as facial expressions and head movements, and spatial arrangement to differentiate and connect clauses. The spatial and visual nature of sign languages provides a unique modality for representing the semantic relationships between clauses, with the physical space around the signer being utilized to set apart or link different parts of the discourse. These methods of clause combining underscore the linguistic sophistication of sign languages, enabling the construction of detailed and complex narratives that mirror the depth of human thought and experience.

An example of clause combining in ASL might be:

IX-me EAT FINISH, IX-me GO STORE.

Here, two clauses, "IX-me EAT FINISH" and "IX-me GO STORE," are combined to express a sequence of actions. Completing the first action (eating) is a prerequisite for commencing the second action (going to the store). The spatial and temporal markers and using index pointing (IX-me) for subject reference in both clauses facilitate a clear understanding of the action sequence and the relationship between the clauses. This example demonstrates the capacity of sign languages to use spatial organization and manual signs to combine clauses effectively, allowing for the expression of complex, sequenced actions within a unified narrative structure.

2.5 Semantics

Semantics in sign language encompasses the study of meaning within this visual-spatial linguistic modality, addressing how signs convey information, ideas, and concepts. Semantics in sign languages operate on multiple levels, from the lexical meanings of individual signs to the complex interpretations of phrases and sentences within broader discourse contexts.

The semantic field in sign languages is rich and varied, incorporating iconicity, where the form of a sign can resemble its meaning alongside arbitrary signs whose meanings are established by convention rather than resemblance. The role of classifiers, spatial grammar, and non-manual signals (such as facial expressions and body posture) adds layers of meaning, enabling sign languages to express nuances of action, emotion, and spatial relationships with precision. Moreover, the dynamic use of signing space allows for the expression of temporal and aspectual nuances and the representation of multiple perspectives and spatial orientations, enhancing the depth and flexibility of semantic interpretation. Through these means, sign languages facilitate a multifaceted communication system that is both expressive and efficient, capable of conveying complex semantic networks and relationships that reflect the cognitive and social realities of sign language users.

Sign Meanings

Sign meaning in sign language semantics delves into the interpretation and significance of signs as isolated units and within discourse's syntactic and pragmatic contexts. This aspect of semantics explores how signs represent objects, actions, concepts, and emotions, integrating the inherent meanings of signs and their modified interpretations in varying contexts. The multifaceted nature of sign meaning encompasses denotation—the direct reference of a sign to a concept or object—and connotation, the associated or implied meanings based on cultural and linguistic contexts. Furthermore, sign languages exploit the visual-spatial modality to encode additional semantic layers using classifiers, directional verbs, and spatial arrangements. These can convey relationships, sizes, shapes, and orientations with specificity and nuance. Incorporating non-manual elements such as facial expressions and body posture adds further depth to sign meaning, allowing for the expression of grammatical distinctions, affective states, and emphatic or interrogative modulations. Thus, the semantic system of sign languages is complex and adaptive, enabling signers to communicate a broad spectrum of information and emotional content.

An example of how sign meaning can vary by context might involve the sign for "FLY" (as in the action of flying). In a sentence, the meaning of "FLY" can be influenced by its syntactic role and the non-manual markers used:

- FLY++ (with repeated movement) could denote the continuous flying action, emphasizing the duration.

- FLY (with eyebrows raised and a questioning expression) could turn the statement into a question about the act of flying or someone's ability to fly.
- FLY-FAST (with an intensified movement) emphasizes the speed of the action, modifying the base meaning to convey additional information about the manner of flying.

These variations illustrate how the meaning of a single sign in sign language is not fixed but can shift and expand in response to linguistic and extralinguistic cues.

Polysemy

Polysemy in sign language semantics refers to the phenomenon where a single sign possesses multiple related meanings or interpretations, depending on its use in context. This linguistic feature mirrors polysemy in spoken languages, underscoring the richness and flexibility of sign languages in conveying a wide array of meanings through a single gestural form. The ability of a sign to convey different meanings is not arbitrary but rooted in the conceptual links between these meanings, often reflecting the sign's historical development or the inherent semantic network it belongs to. Polysemy enhances the efficiency and expressiveness of sign languages, allowing signers to use context, non-manual markers, and syntactic structure to disambiguate the intended meaning of polysemous signs. This dynamic aspect of sign language semantics showcases signers' cognitive and contextual adaptability, who skillfully navigate the semantic landscapes of signs to achieve precise and nuanced communication.

An example of polysemy in ASL is the sign "LIGHT." This sign can represent multiple related concepts:

- LIGHT-bright can refer to the physical property of brightness or illumination, such as "The room is very light."
- LIGHT-weight can denote the lack of physical weight, as in "This box is light."

In each case, the conceptual link between the meanings is clear—the properties of being visually bright and physically not heavy share a notion of "lightness" captured by the same sign in ASL. The intended meaning is usually clarified by the context in which the sign is used, accompanying non-manual signals, and the sentence's syntactic structure.

Homonymy

Homonymy in sign language semantics involves signs that share the same form—handshape, movement, location, and orientation—but have distinct, unrelated meanings. This phenomenon is akin to homonymy in spoken languages, where two words sound alike but differ in meaning. In sign languages, the visual-spatial nature of these homonyms creates unique challenges and opportunities for disambiguation, relying heavily on contextual cues, including the surrounding signs, non-manual markers such as facial expressions, and the broader discourse context. Homonymy enriches the lexicon, allowing for a compact use of the signing space and manual features to convey a wide spectrum of meanings. It underscores the importance of context in interpreting sign language, as signers must adeptly navigate these semantic overlaps to ensure clear and effective communication. The existence of homonyms in sign languages highlights their complexity and nuance, reflecting the depth of cognitive processing involved in sign language use and comprehension.

Examples of homonymy in ASL include:

- BANK can represent the financial institution where money is kept or the land alongside a river. In gloss notation, both meanings are described as "BANK," but the intended meaning is clarified through context.
- BAT might refer to the flying mammal or the equipment used in sports like baseball. Again, both would be glossed as "BAT," with the specific interpretation dependent on the communicative context and possibly non-manual markers that accompany the sign.

Iconicity

Iconicity in sign language semantics refers to the meaningful resemblance between the form of a sign and its referent, a characteristic feature that often distinguishes sign languages from spoken languages. This resemblance can be visual, spatial, or even conceptual, allowing signers to exploit the gestural-visual modality to create signs that are intuitively linked to their meanings. Iconicity facilitates learning and recall by leveraging natural associations between sign forms and their semantic content, enhancing cognitive accessibility and semantic intuition. While not all signs in sign languages are iconic, those that play a crucial role in bridging the gap between linguistic expression and the physical or conceptual world. Iconic signs often evolve from gestural representations of objects, actions, or phenomena and, over time, may become more abstract or stylized. However, their original iconic basis remains a foundational element of their semantic character. The presence of iconicity within sign languages highlights their capacity for descriptive richness and immediacy of communication, reflecting the inherently visual-spatial nature of these languages.

Examples of iconicity in ASL include:

- TREE: This sign is often made by extending the arm upward and splaying the fingers to mimic the branches of a tree. The resemblance between the sign's form and the shape of a tree exemplifies iconicity. In gloss notation, it would be noted as "TREE."

- BOOK: Typically signed by holding your hands together as if opening a book, this sign's form visually resembles the action of opening a real book, making the meaning immediately apparent. In gloss, it is represented as "BOOK."

These examples underscore how iconic signs in ASL and other sign languages employ physical resemblance to convey meaning, enhancing these visual languages' expressive and communicative power.

Metaphor

Metaphor in sign language semantics represents a sophisticated linguistic mechanism where signs extend beyond their literal meanings to express abstract ideas, qualities, or relationships by mapping physical and spatial properties onto conceptual domains. This cognitive and linguistic process mirrors metaphorical thinking in spoken languages, highlighting the universality of metaphor as a fundamental aspect of human communication. In sign languages, metaphors often exploit the visual-spatial modality to draw parallels between the physical world and abstract concepts, utilizing the signer's body and the surrounding space as expressive tools. These visual metaphors can make abstract concepts more tangible, facilitating understanding and engagement by anchoring them in the signer's embodied experience and environmental interactions. Using metaphor in sign languages enriches the lexicon with layers of meaning. It demonstrates the creative and adaptive use of visual-spatial resources to navigate complex conceptual landscapes, illustrating the depth and flexibility of sign languages as full-fledged linguistic systems.

An example of a metaphor in ASL involves the concept of "UNDERSTANDING." The sign for "UNDERSTAND" often looks like a lightbulb turning on above the head, metaphorically suggesting the illumination of an idea or the sudden clarity and comprehension of a concept. In gloss notation, this could be represented as "UNDERSTAND." Still, the metaphorical use imbues the sign with a visual representation of the cognitive process of understanding, echoing the "lightbulb moment" metaphor common in English and other languages.

Another metaphorical example is "TIME-FLOWING," which conceptualizes time as a river flowing past the signer. This use of space and movement in front of the signer's body to represent the passage of time metaphorically captures the abstract notion of time visually concretely. This might be expressed in gloss notation as "TIME-FLOWING," indicating the conceptual mapping of time's flow to the physical action of something moving in space.

Metonymy

Metonymy in sign language semantics is a cognitive and linguistic strategy that involves using one aspect of a concept to stand for the concept as a whole or another related concept. This rhetorical figure relies on the solid associative or contextual relationship between the sign used and the concept it represents, facilitating communication through indirect reference. Metonymy is particularly effective in sign languages due to its visual-spatial nature. It allows signers to exploit physical or spatial characteristics of objects, actions, or contexts to evoke broader ideas or entities. This semantic mechanism enriches sign language discourse, enabling signers to convey complex ideas succinctly and vividly by drawing on shared cultural and contextual knowledge. Metonymy in sign languages underscores their capability for nuanced expression and conceptual flexibility, reflecting the dynamic interplay between linguistic form and cognitive processes in visual-spatial modalities.

An example of metonymy in ASL could involve using the sign for "WHITE-HOUSE" to refer not just to the physical building in Washington, D.C., but metonymically to the executive branch of the United States government or the actions of the presidency. In gloss notation, this could be represented simply as "WHITE-HOUSE," but the understanding that it stands for the presidency or the executive branch relies on the contextual and cultural knowledge shared by the interlocutors.

Another instance is using "PAPER" to refer to academic studies, news, or documentation. It relies on the associative relationship between paper as a physical medium and the information or content it typically carries. In gloss, this would appear as "PAPER," with the broader or related concept it evokes being understood from the discourse context.

2.6 Pragmatics

Pragmatics in sign language involves studying how context influences the interpretation of meaning in communication, focusing on how signers use and understand signs beyond their literal semantic content. This linguistic domain examines the interplay between sign language structure, the intentions and assumptions of interlocutors, and the situational context to understand how messages are conveyed and interpreted in social interactions. Pragmatics covers a range of phenomena, including the use of deixis (pointing signs that refer to persons, places, or things within the communicative context), the role of facial expressions and body language in conveying mood, intention, and emphasis, as well as the principles governing conversation, such as turn-taking, politeness strategies, and the implicit rules that guide the coherence and relevance of communicative exchanges. The pragmatic aspect of sign language highlights the adaptability and sensitivity of signers to the communicative context, enabling them to navigate and negotiate meaning in diverse social settings. Through pragmatic cues, signers can imply irony, express politeness, indicate questions, and manage conversational flow, demonstrating sign language communication's dynamic and context-dependent nature. This underscores the complexity of sign languages as fully formed linguistic systems capable of expressing a broad spectrum of human experience and facilitating nuanced social interaction.

Contextual Interpretation

Contextual interpretation in sign language pragmatics is a critical aspect of understanding and generating meaning in communication, where the situational, cultural, or discursive context significantly influences the meaning of signs or sign sequences. This pragmatics facet underscores sign language's flexibility and adaptability to convey nuanced meanings beyond the literal or surface level of signs. Contextual interpretation encompasses the ability of signers to infer unstated information, recognize implied meanings, and adjust their language use according to the interaction's social norms, relationship dynamics, and communicative goals. It also involves understanding how different contexts can alter the interpretation of identical signs, where factors such as the communicative setting, the participants' backgrounds, and the broader societal norms play pivotal roles. Sign languages, with their rich use of visual-spatial modality, non-manual markers, and classifiers, offer signers a wide range of tools to exploit contextual cues effectively, thereby enriching communication with layers of meaning that are inferred from the context.

For example, the sign "THINK" in ASL can be interpreted differently depending on the context. In an academic setting, with a facial expression denoting concentration, "THINK" might imply deep contemplation or consideration of a complex idea. In contrast, the same sign, "THINK," accompanied by a sarcastic facial expression in a casual conversation, could imply skepticism or disbelief towards the preceding statement. This variation in interpretation highlights how context and non-manual signals shape the understanding of signs, enabling signers to express and perceive subtleties of meaning that are not explicitly encoded in the manual sign.

Conversational Maxims

Conversational maxims in sign language pragmatics, akin to those in spoken language contexts, refer to the implicit rules that guide the cooperative nature of communicative exchanges. These maxims, originating from Grice's Cooperative Principle [21], are adapted in sign language interactions to ensure effective, efficient, and socially appropriate communication. They include the maxims of quantity (providing the right amount of information), quality (making contributions that are true and based on evidence), relation (being relevant to the current topic), and manner (being clear and orderly). In sign language, adherence to these maxims involves selecting and organizing manual signs and strategically using non-manual markers, spatial modulation, and turn-taking cues to convey meaning appropriately and coherently. The visual-spatial nature of sign languages adds complexity and richness to applying conversational maxims as signers navigate the pragmatic nuances of their interactions through manual and non-manual means.

For instance, in a conversational exchange, if a signer asks for details about an upcoming event, the response adhering to the maxim of quantity would include all relevant details (time, place, purpose) without overwhelming the asker with unnecessary information. This could be structured in ASL gloss as follows:

EVENT WHEN? [response with appropriate facial expression for inquiry], followed by EVENT SATURDAY, AT PARK, FOR BIRTHDAY, succinctly answering the query with precise, relevant details.

Adherence to the maxim of manner is evident in the straightforward, sequential arrangement of information.

Deictic Signs

Deictic signs are essential linguistic elements that rely on the context of the discourse for their interpretation, anchoring meaning in the immediate communicative situation. These signs are crucial for establishing reference, direction, location, and time within a conversation, serving as gestural pointers that link the linguistic message to its physical or situational context. Deictic signs in sign languages, including pronouns, demonstratives, and locatives, are inherently tied to these languages' spatial and visual nature, with the signer's body and surrounding space acting as the reference points for conveying meaning. The use of eye gaze, body orientation, and pointing gestures are common deictic mechanisms, allowing signers to specify objects, locations, and participants within the communicative event, grounding the conversation in shared spatial and situational awareness. Deictic expressions in sign language facilitate the conveyance of specific information and play a pivotal role in managing turn-taking, establishing discourse cohesion, and navigating the social dynamics of sign language interaction.

For example, using index finger pointing in ASL can serve multiple deictic functions depending on context; if a signer points to a space on their right while discussing plans, as in IX-HERE PARTY, the gesture "IX-HERE" (indexing 'here') deictically establishes a location for the party within the signing space, which can be referred to later in the conversation. Similarly, pointing towards oneself or the listener with the index finger, as in IX-ME (I/me) or IX-YOU (you), establishes the subjects of the conversation deictically, anchoring the discourse in the present communicative context. These deictic signs, integral to the pragmatics of sign language, highlight the importance of the physical and situational context in interpreting and generating meaning within sign language communication.

Register and Style Variation

Register and style variation reflect the adaptability of sign languages to different social contexts, audience expectations, and communicative purposes. These variations manifest in changes to signing speed, clarity, use of space, choice of vocabulary, and the extent of use of non-manual markers to suit formal, informal, educational, or intimate settings. For instance, a formal lecture in ASL might employ a more expansive use of signing space, precise handshapes, and a specific technical vocabulary, contrasting with a casual conversation among friends, which might feature more colloquial signs, relaxed handshapes, and greater use of facial expressions and body language to convey emotion and emphasis. An example of this variation can be seen in the sign for "UNDERSTAND": in a formal educational setting, the sign might be executed with apparent, deliberate movement, whereas in a casual setting, it might be signed more quickly or with a greater degree of facial expression to convey understanding or seek clarification. This flexibility in register and style enables signers to navigate different social situations effectively, demonstrating sign language communication's social and contextual sensitivity.

2.7 Conclusion

In conclusion, exploring the structure of sign language within this chapter has unveiled the intricate and multifaceted nature of sign languages as dynamic communication systems. From the foundational elements of phonology and morphology, which lay the groundwork for the formation and modification of signs, to the complex interplay of syntax, semantics, and pragmatics in constructing and interpreting messages, sign languages demonstrate remarkable depth and flexibility. The examination of linear and nonlinear structures, alongside the utilization of spatial grammar, role shifting, and contextual interpretation, reveals the unique capabilities of sign languages to convey nuanced meanings and engage in sophisticated discourse. Furthermore, discussing conversational maxims, deictic signs, and variations in register and style highlights the adaptive nature of sign languages to different communicative contexts and social settings.

Quiz Time

1. What is the primary focus of phonology in sign languages?

(A) The study of grammatical rules
(B) The study of meaningful units of signs
(C) The study of sentence structure

2. Which element is not a component of the phonology of sign languages?

(A) Hand shapes
(B) Facial expressions
(C) Vocal intonations

3. What does morphology in sign language analyze?

(A) Sentence formation
(B) The internal structure of signs
(C) The role of facial expressions

4. Which of the following is an example of derivational morphology in sign language?

(A) Changing a sign to indicate tense
(B) Creating new words from existing signs
(C) Using facial expressions to modify meaning

5. What does the process morpheme in the sign for "CHAIR" signify?

(A) A change in handshape
(B) A modification in movement
(C) A facial expression

6. What is fingerspelling used for in sign languages?

(A) To spell out words for which there are no signs
(B) To create new sign language grammar
(C) To replace complex signs with simpler ones

7. What does compounding in sign language involve?

(A) Combining two or more signs to create a new sign
(B) Modifying a sign to express different grammatical features
(C) Using non-manual markers to alter meaning

8. What role do classifiers in sign language play?

(A) They indicate grammatical number and tense
(B) They provide specific information about actions, locations, and characteristics
(C) They define the syntax of the sentence

9. Which method is not used to express inflection in sign language?

(A) Modifying movement to indicate different grammatical categories
(B) Changing the location of the sign
(C) Altering the voice tone

10. What is the role of facial expressions in sign languages?

(A) They are solely used to convey emotions
(B) They are integral to grammar and lexicon
(C) They are rarely used in formal communication

References

1. Corina, D., Sandler, W.: On the nature of phonological structure in sign language. Phonology. 10, 165–207 (1993). https://doi.org/10.1017/S0952675700000038.
2. van der Kooij, E., Crasborn, O.: Syllables and the word-prosodic system in Sign Language of the Netherlands. Lingua. 118, 1307–1327 (2008). https://doi.org/10.1016/j.lingua.2007.09.013.
3. G. Mathur: The morphology-phonology interface in signed languages. (2000).

4. Hulst, H., Kooij, E.: Phonetic implementation and phonetic pre-specification in sign language phonology. In: Goldstein, L., Whalen, D.H., and Best, C.T. (eds.) Laboratory Phonology 8. pp. 265–286. Mouton de Gruyter (2006). https://doi.org/10.1515/9783110197211.1.265.
5. Johnston, T.: Sign Language: Morphology. In: Brown, K. (ed.) Encyclopedia of Language & Linguistics (Second Edition). pp. 324–328. Elsevier, Oxford (2006). https://doi.org/10.1016/B0-08-044854-2/00233-9.
6. Aronoff, M., Meir, I., Sandler, W.: The Paradox of Sign Language Morphology. Language. 81, 301–344 (2005).
7. Napoli, D.J.: Morphological Theory and Sign Languages. In: Audring, J. and Masini, F. (eds.) The Oxford Handbook of Morphological Theory. pp. 593–614. Oxford University Press (2018). https://doi.org/10.1093/oxfordhb/9780199668984.013.37.
8. Mathur, G., Rathmann, C.: Two Types of Non-concatenative Morphology in Signed Languages. In: Deaf around the World. pp. 54–82. Oxford University Press (2010).
9. Lepic, R., Occhino, C.: A Construction Morphology Approach to Sign Language Analysis. In: The Construction of Words. pp. 141–172. Springer International Publishing (2018).
10. Abner, N.: There once was a verb: The predicative core of possessive and nominalization structures in American Sign Language. SL&L. 17, 109–118 (2014). https://doi.org/10.1075/sll.17.1.06abn.
11. Poizner, H., Newkirk, D., Bellugi, U., Klima, E.S.: Representation of inflected signs from American Sign Language in short-term memory. Mem Cogn. 9, 121–131 (1981). https://doi.org/10.3758/BF03202326.
12. Crandall, K.E.: Inflectional Morphemes in the Manual English of Young Hearing-Impaired Children and Their Mothers. Journal of Speech and Hearing Research. 21, 372–386 (1978). https://doi.org/10.1044/jshr.2102.372.
13. Fernald, T.B., Napoli, D.J.: Exploitation of morphological possibilities in signed languages: Comparison of American Sign Language with English. SL&L. 3, 3–58 (2000). https://doi.org/10.1075/sll.3.1.03fer.
14. Perniss, P., Özyürek, A., Morgan, G.: The Influence of the Visual Modality on Language Structure and Conventionalization: Insights From Sign Language and Gesture. Topics in Cognitive Science. 7, 2–11 (2015). https://doi.org/10.1111/tops.12127.
15. Corina, D.P., Jose-Robertson, L.S., Guillemin, A., High, J., Braun, A.R.: Language Lateralization in a Bimanual Language. Journal of Cognitive Neuroscience. 15, 718–730 (2003). https://doi.org/10.1162/jocn.2003.15.5.718.
16. Sandler, W., Lillo-Martin, D.: Sign Language and Linguistic Universals. Cambridge University Press, Cambridge (2006). https://doi.org/10.1017/CBO9781139163910.
17. Lichtenauer, J., Hendriks, E., Reinders, M.: Learning to recognize a sign from a single example. In: 2008 8th IEEE International Conference on Automatic Face & Gesture Recognition. pp. 1–6. IEEE, Amsterdam, Netherlands (2008). https://doi.org/10.1109/AFGR.2008.4813450.
18. Krebs, J., Malaia, E., Wilbur, R.B., Roehm, D.: Psycholinguistic mechanisms of classifier processing in sign language. Journal of Experimental Psychology: Learning, Memory, and Cognition. 47, 998–1011 (2021). https://doi.org/10.1037/xlm0000958.
19. Cogill-Koez, D.: A model of signed language classifier predicates as templated visual representation. SL&L. 3, 209–236 (2000). https://doi.org/10.1075/sll.3.2.04cog.
20. Koenders, E.: Noun classifiers in Hong Kong Sign Language. SL&L. (2024). https://doi.org/10.1075/sll.22004.koe.
21. Davies, B.L.: Grice's Cooperative Principle: Meaning and rationality. Journal of Pragmatics. 39, 2308–2331 (2007). https://doi.org/10.1016/j.pragma.2007.09.002.

Chapter 3
Sign Language Varieties Around the World

3.1 Introduction

The world is a mosaic of languages and cultures, each contributing its distinct hue to the global tapestry of human communication. Within this vibrant expanse, sign languages emerge as a captivating domain, brimming with diversity, history, and cultural significance. Contrary to common misconception, no singular, universal sign language is understood by all deaf individuals worldwide, as explained in the previous chapter. Instead, many sign languages exist, and an estimated 200 different sign languages, each rooted in its community, history, and linguistic landscape. Some of them are listed in Table 3.1 as an example.

The table provides an overview of various sign languages used around the world. It lists 17 different sign languages, each with a corresponding acronym, and the regions where they are predominantly used. ASL is noted for being used in North America, West Africa, and parts of Western Asia.

This chapter explores the diverse array of global sign languages, ranging from urban to indigenous settings. It acknowledges the prominence and extensive research associated with ASL, inviting examination into the vast spectrum of existing sign languages. This includes the distinctive qualities of Arabic Sign Language and the community-driven nature of International Sign Language, each reflecting the unique narrative of its people. A central theme that will be apparent throughout this linguistic survey is the resilience of deaf communities. These communities are the originators and cultivators of sign languages, playing an active and essential role in their development, maintenance, and dissemination.

A. Othman, *Sign Language Processing*,
https://doi.org/10.1007/978-3-031-68763-1_3

Table 3.1 A selection of sign languages around the world

Sign language	Acronym	Country/community
American Sign Language	ASL	North America, West Africa, parts of Western Asia
Black American Sign Language (an ASL dialect)	BASL	African Americans in the United States
French Sign Language	LSF	France
Russian Sign Language	RSL	Russia
Kazakh Sign Language (an RSL Dialect)	KSL	Kazakhstan
Danish Sign Language	DSL	Denmark
Swedish Sign Language	SSL	Sweden
Arab Sign Language Family	ArSL	Example of Subdivisions: – Tunisian Sign Language (LST): Tunisia – Qatari Sign Language (QSL): Qatar – Levantine Arabic Sign Language: Levant region – Egyptian Sign Language: Egypt
South African Sign Language	SASL	South Africa
Indo-Pakistani Sign Language	IPSL	South Asia (India, Pakistan, Nepal, Bangladesh, …)
Chinese Sign Language	CSL	China
Taiwan Sign Language	TSL	Taiwan
Japanese Sign Language	JSL	Japan
British Sign Language	BSL	United Kingdom
Quebec Sign Language	LSQ	Francophone Canada (Mainly Quebec Canada)
Italian Sign Language	LIS	Italy
Dutch Sign Language	NGT	Netherlands
Flemish Sign Language	VGT	Belgium

3.2 International Sign

International Sign (IS) and not International Sign Language, often known as Gestuno, is a form of sign language that is used by the deaf community on an international level, particularly in global meetings by the United Nations, sports events like the Deaflympics, and conferences such as those organized by the World Federation of the Deaf. Unlike other sign languages, it is not associated with a specific country or region but serves as a lingua franca, enabling communication between deaf individuals from different language backgrounds. IS comprises a lexicon of signs agreed upon by the international community and often incorporates elements from various sign languages to maximize understandability across diverse cultural boundaries.

The grammar and vocabulary are simplified to facilitate mutual comprehension and effective communication among deaf individuals globally. The existence and use of IS underscore the adaptability and collaborative spirit of the deaf community, demonstrating their capacity to bridge linguistic gaps and foster inclusivity in international settings [1]. Despite its utility, International Sign is not considered a natural language, but rather a pidgin—a simplified, auxiliary language that develops in multilingual environments for the purpose n between speakers of different native languages [2].

3.3 American Sign Language

American Sign Language, commonly abbreviated ASL, is one of the most prominent and extensively researched sign languages globally. Born from a confluence of historical and societal influences, ASL has become the primary language of many deaf and hard-of-hearing individuals in the United States and parts of Canada. Figure 3.1 showcase countries that are using ASL by the deaf community.

Historical Origins

The history of American Sign Language is complex and evolving, with its origins traced back to the intermixing of local sign languages and French Sign Language [3]. The language has undergone significant historical change, with signs shifting towards arbitrariness rather than maintaining iconicity [4]. The development of ASL has been influenced by the educational system and the Deaf community, leading to its evolution along racial lines and in response to societal pressures [5]. The language is also related to Plains Indian Sign Language, developed and used

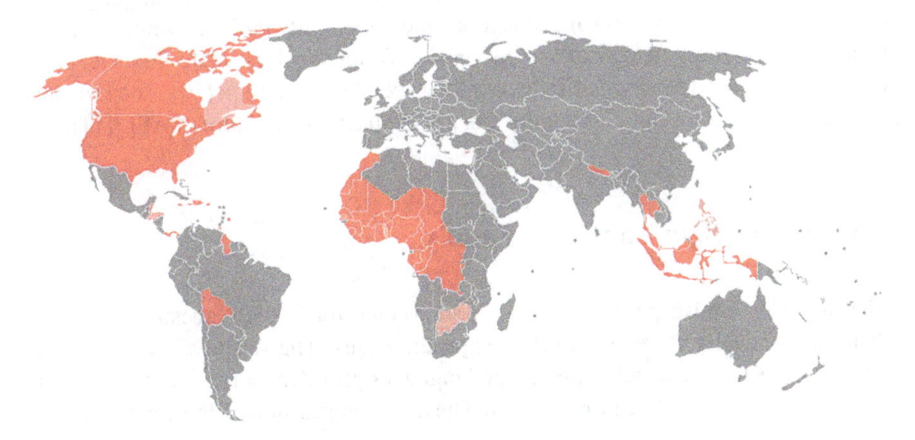

Fig. 3.1 American Sign Language around the world (Image from https://en.wikipedia.org/wiki/American_Sign_Language (CC BY-SA 3.0))

primarily by hearing people [6]. Despite these influences, ASL has emerged as a rich, complex, and mature language.

Linguistic Features

Like other sign languages, ASL boasts a rich phonological and morphological structure. It utilizes handshapes, facial expressions, and body movements to convey meaning, and its syntax can often differ significantly from English. For instance, the ASL sentence structure might employ a "*topic-comment*" format, also known as "topicalization," which differs from the typical English subject-verb-object pattern [7]. For example, the sentence "The girl loves chocolate" is signed as follow:

GIRL^{topic} CHOCOLATE LOVE

Variations, Dialects and Societal Influence

ASL is not monolithic. Over time and across different regions and communities, variations and dialects of ASL have emerged. Regional influences, racial and ethnic identities, and educational backgrounds can contribute to these variations, making ASL a diverse language [8]. For example, Black American Sign Language (BASL) is a dialect of ASL commonly used by deaf African Americans in the United States. Tactile ASL (TASL) is a variety of ASL used throughout the United States by and with the deaf-blind.[1]

ASL is intrinsically tied to the cultural identity of the American Deaf community. Through ASL, narratives, poetry, and performances have been crafted, reflecting the community's experiences, challenges, and triumphs. The language has played a pivotal role in activism, education, and community building, reinforcing its significance beyond mere communication [9]. Various factors, including age, education, and cultural awareness, influenced the social construction [10]. The size and homogeneity of the Deaf community can also impact the structure of ASL [11].

3.4 Arabic Sign Language Family

The linguistic landscape of the Arab world, known for its rich tapestry of spoken dialects, is equally diverse regarding sign languages. The Arabic Sign Language family comprises a constellation of sign languages prevalent across the Arab world, exhibiting a variety of regional forms. These languages mirror the linguistic and

[1] The deaf-blind manual alphabet: https://www.deafblind.com/card.html

cultural diversity of the Middle East and North Africa (Fig. 3.2), with each regional variant reflecting its unique lexical and syntactic patterns influenced by local dialects and traditions.

For instance, Levantine Arabic Sign Language shows variances that correlate with the spoken Levantine Arabic dialects, while Egyptian Sign Language incorporates elements specific to Egyptian culture and spoken language. The emergence and evolution of these sign languages are products of intricate social interactions within deaf communities, where shared experiences and regional identity consolidate to form distinct communicative systems. Although these languages share some commonalities due to the overarching influence of Arabic culture, they are as distinct from each other as the spoken languages in their respective regions. The recognition and study of the Arabic Sign Language family are critical for appreciating the nuances of regional deaf cultures and for developing inclusive linguistic policies that address the communicative needs of the deaf in the Arab world.

Unified Arabic Signs

An ongoing effort has been establishing a set of Unified Arabic Signs for decades. This initiative aims to harmonize communication among deaf individuals across the Arab world by creating a standardized lexicon of signs that would be widely recognized and understood, notwithstanding regional variations. Such efforts are often seen as parallel to the modern standardization of Arabic for the spoken and written language, aiming to facilitate more precise and more efficient interactions in educational, social, and possibly official settings. The efforts to unify sign language signs across the Arabic-speaking world involves careful consideration of cultural

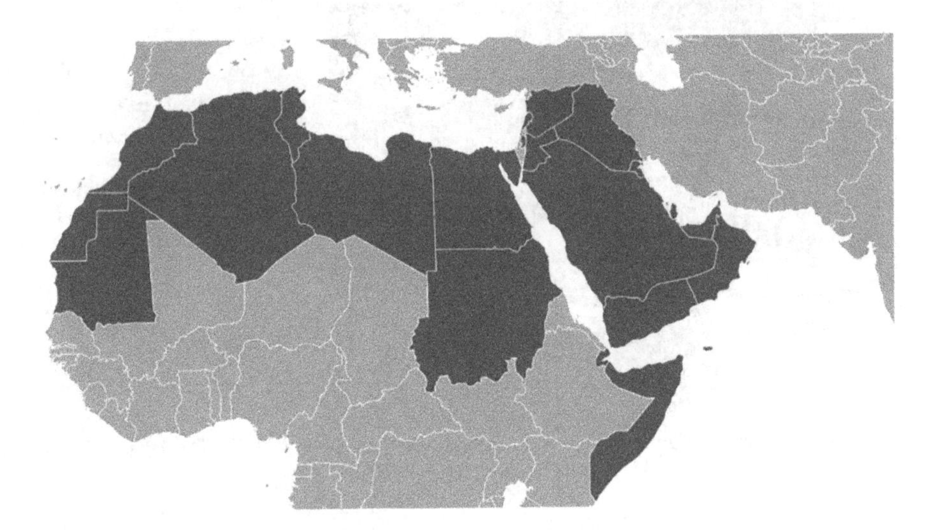

Fig. 3.2 List of Arab countries

appropriateness and linguistic feasibility, considering the need to respect the distinctiveness of local sign languages while striving for a cohesive system that promotes connectivity and inclusivity. Through conferences, collaborative workshops, and scholarly exchanges, experts in sign linguistics and community representatives engage in the meticulous process of selecting and codifying signs, which involves empirical studies and consensus-building to ensure that the unified signs are representative and functional.

For example, in Algeria and Tunisia, sign languages are influenced by the French Sign Language due to colonization. However, Egyptian and Jordanian Sign Languages have distinct lexicons and structures, although they share some similarities due to cultural exchanges [12].

Figures 3.3 and 3.4 present efforts conducted by the Arab League and the State of Qatar to unify domain-specific signs for the Arab deaf communities. This initiative seeks to establish a standardized set of signs that can be universally understood across the Arab world, enhancing inter-regional communication and promoting a cohesive identity among deaf communities [13].

Challenges and Controversies

While the concept of unified signs is noble in intent, it faces challenges. Standardization can sometimes overlook regional nuances and cultural significances, leading to a loss of rich linguistic diversity. Moreover, top-down initiatives might not always resonate at the grassroots level, where regional sign languages have been deeply entrenched and evolved over generations [14].

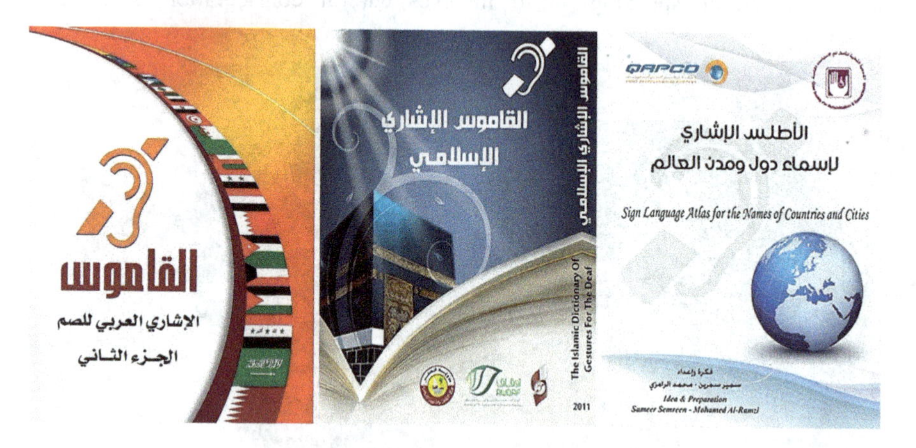

Fig. 3.3 From left to right: (1) The Arabic Signs Dictionary—Part 2 (2) The Islamic Signs Dictionary (3) The Atlas Signs for country and cities names

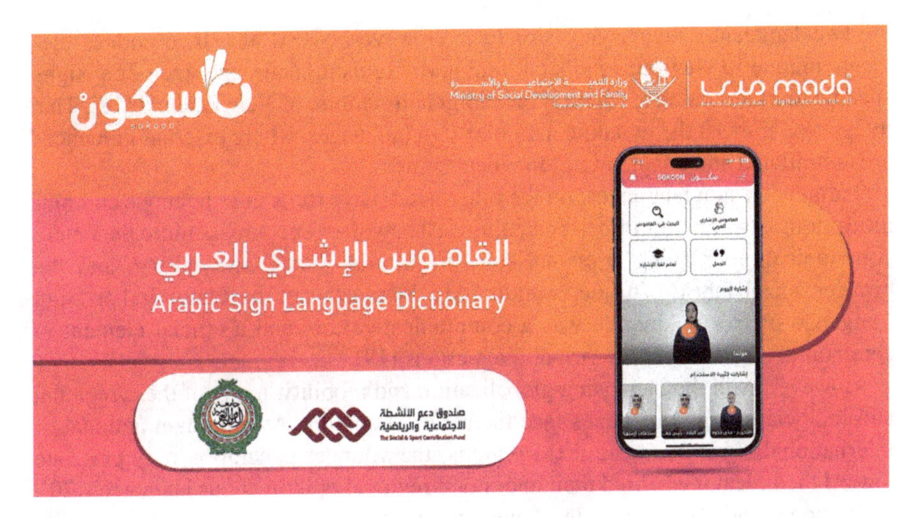

Fig. 3.4 The Arabic Sign Language Dictionary Mobile Application Sokoon, an initiative by the Ministry of Social Development and Family in the State of Qatar

Cultural and Societal Implications

Arabic Sign Languages carry cultural narratives, histories, and values like their spoken counterparts. The signs often encapsulate stories, traditions, and societal norms unique to each region. The balance between preserving these distinct identities and pushing for a unified communication system remains a topic of discussion and research within the Arab deaf communities [15].

The dynamics between Arabic Sign Languages and Unified Signs mirrors, to an extent, the ongoing dialogue between regional spoken Arabic dialects and Modern Standard Arabic. As the discourse progresses, it will be essential to ensure that standardization efforts preserve and celebrate the rich linguistic and cultural diversity inherent in the Arab world's sign languages.

3.5 Regional and Indigenous Sign Languages

Numerous regional and indigenous sign languages lie beyond the well-documented and researched national sign languages such as ASL. These languages, often developed in isolated communities or specific regions, provide a rich tapestry of linguistic diversity, reflecting their communities' unique histories, cultures, and experiences [16].

A notable example of a regional sign language influenced by a national sign language is New Zealand Sign Language (NZSL). NZSL, while a distinct entity, has been significantly influenced by BSL due to Britain's historical colonization of New Zealand [17]. This influence is observed in the similarities between many signs and the two languages' underlying structure. However, NZSL also incorporates elements unique to New Zealand's cultural and linguistic landscape, including signs specific to Maori culture, which is the indigenous culture of New Zealand [18]. This integration mirrors the dynamic nature of sign languages, where external influences are assimilated and adapted to fit the local context.

Indigenous sign languages, on the other hand, have roots in indigenous communities' long-standing traditions and cultures. They often encompass more than mere communication, playing a pivotal role in cultural rituals, storytelling, and the broader social fabric of these communities. For instance, the Plains Indian Sign Language of North America was a communicative tool and a crucial element in ceremonial contexts and intertribal interactions [19].

However, with the increasing globalization and mobility, many of these regional and indigenous sign languages face threats of extinction. As dominant national or international signs permeate these regions, the younger generation may gravitate toward them, leaving behind their ancestors' regional or indigenous languages [20].

Regional and indigenous sign languages are vibrant reminders of the diversity and richness of human linguistic heritage. Their preservation and documentation are not merely academic undertakings but are also crucial for maintaining the cultural and historical identities of the communities they represent.

Considering the sociolinguistic dynamics between national and regional sign languages within deaf communities and acknowledging the broader societal context in which these communities are often viewed through the lens of minority status or disability, an intriguing research question emerges: How do the interactions between national and regional sign languages within deaf communities reflect and influence their social positioning and rights to information access? This question investigates the complex interplay of language, identity, and societal norms, examining how the development and usage of sign languages within and across deaf communities serve as a mechanism for negotiating their status as minority or disabled groups. It invites a multidisciplinary investigation into how linguistic practices in deaf communities contribute to their empowerment or marginalization, particularly about their legal and societal rights to access information. This research could shed light on the potential of sign languages as tools for advocacy and change, challenging prevailing narratives around minority and disability rights.

3.6 The Influence of Deaf Communities on Sign Language Development

Deaf communities, with their rich histories, shared experiences, and cultural dynamics, have played an indomitable role in shaping the trajectory of sign language development. These communities, often bonded by a shared understanding of deafness and the necessity for a visual mode of communication, have been at the forefront of linguistic innovation, preservation, and propagation of sign languages [21, 22].

Historically, sign languages organically sprouted and flourished within the tightly-knit circles of deaf communities. While primarily functional, these languages also emerged as powerful symbols of identity and belonging, allowing members to communicate, narrate stories, and pass on traditions. In places where oral languages predominated, deaf communities became the bastions of sign languages, ensuring their continuity across generations [23].

The establishment of deaf schools and institutions in the nineteenth and twentieth centuries further catalyzed the development and standardization of sign languages. However, it also marked a period where sign languages faced challenges, particularly from oralist movements that sought to promote speech over signing. Despite such adversities, deaf communities held fast, preserving their linguistic heritage and, over time, advocating for its recognition and respect [24, 25].

In contemporary times, deaf communities have been instrumental in advancing research, documentation, and technological innovations related to sign languages. Through collaborations with linguists, educators, and technologists, these communities have facilitated the creation of dictionaries, digital platforms, and educational resources, further enriching the ecosystem of sign language learning and usage [11].

3.7 Cross-Cultural Communication Through Sign Language

Cross-cultural communication through sign language presents unique challenges and opportunities for interaction beyond linguistic boundaries. Unlike spoken languages, sign languages are not mutually intelligible worldwide, which can complicate interactions among deaf individuals from different linguistic backgrounds. However, instances of cross-cultural communication facilitated by sign languages often exemplify the adaptability and resourcefulness of deaf communities in international settings.

One crucial mechanism for cross-cultural communication among deaf communities is International Sign, as previously introduced in Sect. 3.1. IS, a pidgin sign language, plays a significant role at global deaf gatherings. Quinto-Pozos and Mehta's work underscores IS's utility in surmounting communication barriers in such international contexts, though they caution against its limitations in accurately transmitting complex ideas and subtle distinctions [26].

Efforts to navigate language barriers in global settings include fostering shared signs, as evidenced within Arabic Sign Languages, leveraging visual-gestural communication methods, and employing technological aids like video interpreting services to enhance mutual understanding. Nonetheless, the attempt faces persistent hurdles, notably in signs' standardization and preparing interpreters for diverse linguistic and cultural landscape demands.

The heterogeneity of sign languages and their embeddedness in distinct sociocultural milieus are critically examined [27]. Moreover, cross-modal bilingualism, encompassing the concurrent use of signed and spoken languages, is a natural and evolving practice [28]. Additionally, the distinctive linguistic ecosystem of the deaf community, characterized by reliance on International Sign and adaptable communication strategies, is delineated, presenting a comprehensive view of the complexities inherent in cross-cultural exchanges facilitated by sign language [29].

3.8 Preservation of Endangered Sign Languages

The urgency of preserving endangered sign languages has garnered significant attention, necessitating a multifaceted strategy that intertwines documentation, community support, and technological innovation. Jongbloed underscores the critical need for comprehensive documentation as a cornerstone of preservation efforts [30], a sentiment echoed by Braithwaite [31], who calls for increased linguistic intervention to support endangered sign language communities. The introduction of bilingualism and multimedia materials as preservation tools represents a vital strategy for maintaining the vitality of these languages within their communities.

The role of technology, particularly the potential for AI-based tools proposed by Katinskaya et al., marks a pioneering approach to documenting and revitalizing endangered sign languages [32]. Technological advances, including mobile applications and online platforms, and even virtual reality and Metaverse, offer new avenues for sign language preservation. These tools can enhance accessibility to learning resources and create spaces for community interaction and language use.

The combined insights from these researchers point to the necessity of a comprehensive approach that includes recording languages for academic purposes and supporting their active use among native speakers. Developing educational programs that integrate endangered sign languages and using digital platforms for broader engagement is critical for these languages' survival. Efforts to preserve endangered sign languages thus require collaboration across disciplines, leveraging traditional methods and innovative technologies to ensure these languages do not fade into obscurity.

Several notable projects have been initiated worldwide to document and revitalize endangered sign languages, similar to Sokoon App conducted by the Ministry of Social Development and Family in Qatar presented in Fig. 3.4, showcasing the commitment of various organizations and communities to preserving this vital aspect of cultural heritage. Here are some examples:

- **LAR (Endangered Languages Archive) at SOAS University of London:**[2] ELAR hosts a collection of materials from endangered languages around the world, including sign languages. The archive makes these resources available to

[2] Endangered Languages Archive Repository: https://glocal.soas.ac.uk/endangered-languages-archive/

communities, researchers, and the public to support language preservation and revitalization efforts.

- **Sign Language Documentation Training Center in India:**[3] Established by the Indian Sign Language Research and Training Centre (ISLRTC), this initiative focuses on training individuals in sign language documentation techniques. The goal is to create a repository of Indian Sign Languages, including endangered dialects, to support research, teaching, and the preservation of linguistic diversity within the deaf community.
- **"Sign-Hub" Project:**[4] Preserving, Researching, and Fostering the Linguistic, Historical, and Cultural Heritage of European Deaf Signing Communities with an Integral Resource funded by the European Commission. This project aims to document and preserve the sign languages of several European countries, focusing particularly on those that are less known or at risk of disappearing. It includes creating archives, developing grammars, and producing dictionaries for these languages.

3.9 The Role of Sign Language Interpreters

The profession of sign language interpreting plays a crucial role in facilitating communication between deaf, hard-of-hearing, and hearing individuals, bridging linguistic and cultural gaps across diverse settings. This profession requires unique skills, encompassing linguistic proficiency, cultural competence, and ethical integrity. Becoming a sign language interpreter typically involves rigorous training, certification processes, adherence to ethical standards, and navigating the intricate challenges of interpreting across modalities.

Training for sign language interpreters often begins with comprehensive language learning, including both the target sign language and the spoken language(s) in the interpreter's region. Educational programs may range from diploma to degree levels, offering courses in linguistics, deaf culture, interpreting techniques, and practical interpreting experiences. Upon formal education, aspiring interpreters must undergo certification processes, which vary by country and may include written exams, performance assessments, and continuing education requirements. For example, in the United States, the Registry of Interpreters for the Deaf (RID) offers several certification options, each tailored to different interpreting settings.

Sign language interpreters are bound by professional codes of ethics designed to uphold the dignity and rights of all parties involved in the communication process. These ethical standards emphasize confidentiality, impartiality, accuracy, and respect for cultural diversity. Interpreters must navigate complex moral dilemmas, balancing their role as neutral facilitators of communication with the need to act in

[3] Sign Language Documentation Training Center in India: https://www.islrtc.nic.in/

[4] SignHub: https://www.uva.nl/en/discipline/sign-linguistics/research/sign-hub/

the best interest of their clients. Professional development and ethical training engagement are essential for interpreters to stay aligned with best practices and evolving standards.

Interpreting between spoken and sign languages presents various challenges, from linguistic differences to cultural nuances. Sign languages are visually oriented, employing space, gestures, and facial expressions to convey meaning, which differs fundamentally from spoken languages' auditory and sequential nature. Interpreters must adeptly transform spoken language into its visual-spatial counterpart and vice versa, often requiring creative solutions to accurately express idiomatic phrases, technical terms, and cultural references.

Cultural competence is another critical aspect of sign language interpreting. Deaf cultures have norms, values, and communication styles, which interpreters must understand and respect. This cultural knowledge enables interpreters to provide more accurate and contextually appropriate interpretations, facilitating a deeper understanding and interaction between parties.

3.10 Sign Language Recognition and Legal Status

The legal recognition of sign languages in various countries marks a significant advancement in the rights and societal inclusion of deaf communities. This recognition often comes in legislation or amendments to existing laws, ensuring that sign languages are afforded the same status as spoken languages within a country. Such legal frameworks can profoundly impact the deaf community by guaranteeing access to education, media, and public services in their native sign language.

In education, legal recognition of sign languages can mandate the inclusion of sign language as a medium of instruction for deaf students. This approach not only supports the linguistic development of deaf children but also affirms their cultural identity and rights to education in their first language. For instance, the United States' Individuals with Disabilities Education Act (IDEA) requires that students with disabilities, including those who are deaf or hard of hearing, receive a free appropriate public education in the least restrictive environment, which may include instruction in ASL.

Some countries have introduced legislation requiring television broadcasters to provide sign language interpretation or subtitles for deaf and hard-of-hearing viewers. The United Kingdom, under the Communications Act 2003, mandates that a certain percentage of television programming must be accessible through sign language interpretation, closed captioning, or audio description, thereby enhancing media accessibility for the deaf community.

Public services and governmental communications also fall under the purview of such legislation. Countries like Finland, through the Finnish Sign Language Act, have recognized Finnish Sign Language and Finland-Swedish Sign Language as their own right, guaranteeing the deaf community the right to use sign language and receive information in sign language in dealings with government agencies and courts.

The legal recognition of sign languages strengthens the civil rights of deaf individuals by acknowledging their language and cultural identity. It empowers deaf communities by ensuring equal opportunities to participate in all aspects of societal life, from education and employment to political processes and healthcare. Legal recognition can lead to establishing interpreter services, developing educational curricula in sign language, and producing sign language media content, thereby enhancing the visibility and acceptance of sign languages in mainstream society.

Moreover, such legal frameworks contribute to breaking down communication barriers and fostering a more inclusive environment for deaf individuals. They underscore the importance of linguistic diversity and the need to protect minority languages as a matter of cultural heritage and human rights. However, the implementation of these laws varies, and continuous advocacy is often necessary to ensure that the rights afforded by legal recognition are fully realized in practice. The government's commitment to enforcing these laws and allocating resources for their implementation is crucial for their success.

3.11 Conclusion

In conclusion, this chapter has traversed the multifaceted landscape of sign language varieties worldwide, shedding light on the rich tapestry of linguistic diversity within deaf communities. From the widespread use of American Sign Language across continents to the nuanced regional variations within the Arab Sign Language family, it is evident that sign languages are as diverse and complex as spoken languages, each embedded within its unique cultural and historical context.

The exploration of International Sign underscored its role as a lingua franca among deaf individuals at international gatherings, facilitating cross-cultural communication and fostering a global deaf identity. However, the challenges and limitations of IS also highlight the need for further research and development to enhance its efficacy as a tool for international dialogue.

The documentation and preservation of endangered sign languages have emerged as a critical area of concern. Initiatives such as the Sign-Hub project and efforts by the Ministry of Social Development and Family in Qatar exemplify the global commitment to safeguarding these languages for future generations. These actions not only preserve linguistic diversity but also ensure that the cultural and historical narratives of deaf communities are not lost.

Sign language interpreters are integral to bridging communication gaps between deaf and hearing individuals. The training, certification, and ethical considerations associated with the profession underscore the complexity of this vital service. Moreover, the legal recognition of sign languages in various countries represents a significant advancement in deaf rights, mandating access to education, media, and public services in sign language and enhancing the overall quality of life for deaf individuals.

This chapter has attempted to provide a comprehensive overview of the world's sign languages, illustrating the vibrancy and resilience of deaf communities. It emphasizes the importance of recognizing, respecting, and supporting the linguistic rights of deaf individuals, advocating for an inclusive society where sign languages are celebrated and preserved. As we continue to advance our understanding of sign languages and their impact on the deaf community, it is crucial to engage in ongoing dialogue, research, and advocacy to ensure that the diversity of human language, in all its forms, is recognized and valued.

Quiz Time

1. What is the International Sign often used for?

(A) Local community events
(B) International meetings and events
(C) Everyday communication in the Deaf community

2. Which of the following is not true about American Sign Language (ASL)?

(A) It is used primarily in the United States and Canada.
(B) It is influenced by French Sign Language (LSF).
(C) It is the same as British Sign Language (BSL).

3. What does the Arabic Sign Language family reflect?

(A) A uniform set of signs used across the Arab world
(B) The linguistic and cultural diversity of the Middle East and North Africa
(C) A single standardized sign language

4. Which sign language is known for its use among African Americans in the United States?

(A) Black American Sign Language (BASL)
(B) American Sign Language (ASL)
(C) French Sign Language (LSF)

5. What is a primary function of International Sign?

(A) To replace local sign languages
(B) To serve as a pidgin for basic communication at international events
(C) To be the global standard for all sign language communication

6. What challenges does the standardization of sign languages, such as Unified Arabic Signs, face?

(A) It is universally accepted without controversies
(B) It may overlook regional nuances and cultural significance
(C) It makes sign languages more uncomplicated to learn globally

7. Which region's sign language was influenced by British historical colonization?

(A) American Sign Language
(B) New Zealand Sign Language (NZSL)
(C) Indo-Pakistani Sign Language

8. What role do regional and indigenous sign languages play beyond communication?

(A) They serve no additional purpose.
(B) They are used in educational contexts only.
(C) They play a role in cultural rituals and social interactions.

9. Which initiative aims to create a standardized lexicon of signs across the Arab world?

(A) The European Commission's Sign Language Project
(B) Unified Arabic Signs initiative
(C) Global Sign Language Rights

10. What is noted about the Arabic Sign Language family about spoken languages?

(A) They are less complex than spoken languages
(B) They mirror the diversity of spoken dialects across the region
(C) They are becoming less popular

References

1. Emmorey, K., Reilly, J.S. eds: Language, Gesture, and Space. Psychology Press (2013). https://doi.org/10.4324/9780203773413.
2. Rosenstock, R.: The role of iconicity in International Sign. Sign Language Studies. 8, 131–159 (2008).
3. Caron, D.B.: American Sign Language. 113–114 (2008). https://doi.org/10.1002/9780470373699.speced0117.
4. Frishberg, N.: Arbitrariness and Iconicity: Historical Change in American Sign Language. Language. 51, 696 (1975). https://doi.org/10.2307/412894.
5. Significant gestures: a history of American Sign Language. Choice Reviews Online. 44, 44-5118-44–5118 (2007). https://doi.org/10.5860/CHOICE.44-5118.
6. Armstrong, D.F.: Hand Talk: Sign Language among American Indian Nations (review). sls. 12, 155–157 (2011). https://doi.org/10.1353/sls.2011.0018.
7. Valli, C., Lucas, C.: Linguistics of American sign language: An introduction. Gallaudet University Press (2000).
8. Bayley, R., Lucas, C., Rose, M.: Variation in American Sign Language: The case of DEAF. Journal of Sociolinguistics. 4, 81–107 (2000). https://doi.org/10.1111/1467-9481.00104.
9. Bauman, H.-D.L.: Open your eyes: Deaf studies talking. U of Minnesota Press (2008).
10. McDermid, C.: Social Construction of American Sign Language--English Interpreters. Journal of Deaf Studies and Deaf Education. 14, 105–130 (2009). https://doi.org/10.1093/deafed/enn012.

11. Meir, I., Israel, A., Sandler, W., Padden, C.A., Aronoff, M.: The influence of community on language structure: Evidence from two young sign languages. LV. 12, 247–291 (2012). https://doi.org/10.1075/lv.12.2.04mei.
12. Hendriks, H.B., Baker, A.: Jordanian Sign Language: Aspects of grammar from a cross-linguistic perspective. LOT PhD dissertation, University of Amsterdam, Utrecht (2008).
13. Al-Fityani, K., Padden, C.: Sign language geography in the Arab world. Sign languages: A Cambridge survey. 20, (2010).
14. Brevik, J.-K.: Deaf identities in the making: Local lives, transnational connections. Gallaudet University Press (2005).
15. Owens, J.: Arabic sociolinguistics. Arabica. 48, 419–469 (2001).
16. Nonaka, A.M.: The forgotten endangered languages: Lessons on the importance of remembering from Thailand's Ban Khor Sign Language. Language in society. 33, 737–767 (2004).
17. Schembri, A., McKee, D., McKee, R., Pivac, S., Johnston, T., Goswell, D.: Phonological variation and change in Australian and New Zealand Sign Languages: The location variable. Lang Var Change. 21, 193–231 (2009). https://doi.org/10.1017/S0954394509990081.
18. Simchowitz, M.: Language practices of Māori Deaf New Zealand Sign Language users for identity expression, https://openaccess.wgtn.ac.nz/articles/thesis/Language_practices_of_M_ori_Deaf_New_Zealand_Sign_Language_users_for_identity_expression/22798976, (2023).
19. Farnell, B.M.: Do you see what I mean?: Plains Indian sign talk and the embodiment of action. University of Texas Press (1995).
20. Kusters, A.: Deaf Utopias? Reviewing the Sociocultural Literature on the World's "Martha's Vineyard Situations." Journal of deaf studies and deaf education. 15, 3–16 (2010).
21. Ladd, D.P.: Understanding Deaf Culture: In Search of Deafhood. Multilingual Matters, Clevedon, England ; Buffalo (2003).
22. Ladd, P., Lane, H.: Deaf ethnicity, deafhood, and their relationship. Sign Language Studies. 13, 565–579 (2013).
23. Sutton-Spence, R., Woll, B.: The linguistics of British Sign Language: an introduction. Cambridge University Press (1999).
24. Padden, C., Humphries, T.: Inside Deaf Culture. Harvard University Press (2005). https://doi.org/10.2307/j.ctvjz83v3.
25. Rosen, R.S.: Looking inside or outside? A review of inside deaf culture, https://academic.oup.com/jdsde/article-abstract/12/3/406/490078, (2007).
26. Marschark, M.: Sign language interpreting and interpreter education: Directions for research and practice. Oxford University Press (2005).
27. Zeshan, U.: Sign Languages of the World. In: Encyclopedia of Language & Linguistics. pp. 358–365. Elsevier (2006). https://doi.org/10.1016/B0-08-044854-2/00243-1.
28. Menéndez, B.: Cross-modal bilingualism: language contact as evidence of linguistic transfer in sign bilingual education. International Journal of Bilingual Education and Bilingualism. 13, 201–223 (2010). https://doi.org/10.1080/13670050903474101.
29. Hiddinga, A., Crasborn, O.: Signed languages and globalization. Lang. Soc. 40, 483–505 (2011). https://doi.org/10.1017/S0047404511000480.
30. Uribe-Jongbloed, E.: Endangered languages: Heritage of humanity in dire need of protection Four approaches which support their preservation and maintenance. Revista Folios. 65 (2017). https://doi.org/10.17227/01234870.26folios65.70.
31. Braithwaite, B.: Sign language endangerment and linguistic diversity. Language. 95, e161–e187 (2019). https://doi.org/10.1353/lan.2019.0025.
32. Katinskaia, A., Yangarber, R.: Digital Cultural Heritage and Revitalization of Endangered Finno-Ugric Languages. In: DHN. pp. 111–121 (2018).

Chapter 4
Sign Language Acquisition and Education

4.1 Introduction

The linguistic domain is profoundly shaped by its intrinsic structure and the methodologies through which it is assimilated, internalized, and disseminated. Sign languages, distinguished by their unique visual-spatial modality, present an intriguing perspective on the interrelationship among cognitive processes, cultural influences, and pedagogical strategies. This chapter dips into this nexus, offering an exhaustive analysis of the nuances of sign language acquisition and the pedagogical frameworks that support its instruction.

The process of acquiring sign language, whether as a first or subsequent language, is a complex task as discussed in previous chapters, influenced by a spectrum of factors from individual cognitive capacities to broader societal and cultural contexts. This exploration into the developmental benchmarks of deaf children who adopt sign language as their primary means of communication provides insights into both the universal and distinct aspects of language learning mechanisms. Similarly, the study of individuals learning sign language as an additional language offers a fascinating glimpse into their adaptation process, highlighting the challenges they face and the parallels they draw from their prior linguistic experiences. Beyond acquisition, the narrative extends to learning methodologies designed explicitly for sign languages, incorporating established educational theories and innovative practices. This chapter illuminates effective pedagogical strategies, from classroom engagement techniques to curriculum design, ensuring proficient language acquisition outcomes.

In the contemporary era, technological advancements have significantly influenced virtually every facet of human existence, including sign language education. The digital revolution has ushered in many tools and platforms that have redefined the modalities through which sign languages are taught, learned, and utilized. These technological interventions, ranging from interactive online courses to immersive

A. Othman, *Sign Language Processing*,
https://doi.org/10.1007/978-3-031-68763-1_4

virtual realities like Metaverse, have augmented the dynamism of sign language instruction, extending its reach to a global audience irrespective of geographical constraints.

This chapter elucidates the methodologies involved in the acquisition and learning of sign languages. It explores the diverse strategies individuals employ to adapt, innovate, and persevere in their quest for effective communication from different environments and ecosystems.

4.2 First Language Acquisition in Deaf Children

The first language acquisition process in deaf children presents a unique avenue for understanding the intersection of language development, cognitive psychology, and neurobiology. Unlike their hearing counterparts, deaf children often acquire language in a visual-spatial rather than auditory-oral modality. This difference fundamentally alters the trajectory and mechanisms of language acquisition, providing valuable insights into the flexibility and resilience of the human language faculty.

Sign languages are natural languages with unique structures and rules that children readily acquire [1]. They share vital linguistic properties with spoken languages, such as phonological and morphosyntactic structural levels, and are primarily controlled by the brain's left hemisphere, as explained in Chap. 3. The study of sign languages has contributed significantly to our understanding of human language, and its investigation raises fundamental questions about human language capacity [2]. They have also provided valuable insights into the human capacity for language, particularly in the context of the brain's processing of language [3, 4]. Furthermore, the investigation of sign languages has contributed to the development of a general model of human language, Universal Grammar (UG) [5]. However, the graphical representation of sign languages with various transcription systems remains challenging [6].

Like spoken language, early exposure to sign language is critical for optimal language development in deaf children. Research suggests a sensitive period for language acquisition, particularly during the first few years of life. Hurford supported the existence of a sensitive period for language acquisition, suggesting that this period ends around puberty [7]. This is further corroborated by Ruben [8], who identified specific time frames for critical and sensitive periods of language development, including phonology, syntax, and semantics. These studies highlight the importance of early language exposure and acquisition, particularly during the first few years of life. During this time, the brain exhibits heightened plasticity, allowing for efficient acquisition of a language system.

Early exposure to sign language has been shown to improve language development in deaf children significantly [9]. This is further supported by the positive effects of ASL rhyme, rhythm, and handshape awareness activities on deaf children's phonological awareness [10]. Deaf children's high levels of communicative competence, including attention-getting skills, have also been attributed to their early exposure to sign language [11]. Additionally, sign language has been found to empower non-deaf children with communication disabilities, further highlighting its positive impact on language development [12]. Conversely, most deaf children born to hearing parents often experience delayed exposure to sign languages. This delay can result in linguistic, cognitive, and social repercussions, highlighting the critical nature of early and consistent access to a language that is fully accessible to children [13].

The study of first language acquisition in deaf children has theoretical implications for our understanding of language universals, neurocognitive underpinnings of language, and the role of the environment in shaping language development. It challenges traditional notions of language acquisition that are heavily biased toward auditory-oral modalities and underscores the flexibility of the human language faculty. Practically, these insights advocate policies and practices that ensure early and consistent access to sign language in deaf children. They highlighted the necessity of supporting deaf parents and providing resources for hearing parents to learn sign language, thus facilitating optimal linguistic and cognitive development in deaf children.

First, language acquisition in deaf children, characterized by its visual-spatial modality, offers a unique perspective on the nature of human language and cognition. The evidence overwhelmingly supports the importance of early exposure to sign language, the role of social interaction, and the profound impact of these factors on the developmental trajectories of deaf children. Understanding and supporting the linguistic rights and needs of deaf children is a matter of educational policy and a fundamental issue of cognitive and linguistic equity.

4.3 Second Language Acquisition of Sign Languages

The differences between first and second language acquisition are significant, with the latter being a conscious process that often requires more effort and practice [14]. Attitudinal factors, such as the learner's attitude toward the language and its speakers, can also play a crucial role in second language acquisition [15]. While first-language acquisition is often unconscious and occurs naturally, second-language acquisition typically requires more detailed instruction and systematic vocabulary enhancement [16]. Despite these differences, there are parallels between the two, such as the ability of infants and young children to develop speech effortlessly in their first language [17].

Research on acquiring sign language as a second language highlights several unique challenges. Schönström emphasized the need for more sign language acquisition research, given the differences in modality between signed and spoken languages [18]. Mayer discussed the specific difficulties faced by deaf learners in developing English literacy as a second language, mainly due to language proficiency and educational models [19]. Hoiting underscores the gradual transition from gestural to linguistic forms in early sign language acquisition, focusing on managing gaze and communication requirements [20]. Woll points to the increasing interest in sign language and deaf culture, underscoring the importance of bilingualism and sign linguistics [21].

The age at which individuals begin learning a second language significantly affects their proficiency outcomes, especially in sign language. The critical period hypothesis suggests an optimal window for language acquisition, after which the ability to learn a language with a native-like proficiency decline. For sign languages, this period is thought to be even more stringent because of the visuospatial and kinetic nature of the language, which may require more plastic neural circuits that are more flexible at younger ages. Early learners often achieve higher levels of fluency and fewer accents in their sign language abilities than those who start learning later in life. Learners usually transfer elements from their first to second language. In the context of sign language acquisition, this can manifest in several ways depending on the learner's language rank. For hearing learners with spoken language as their first language, the transfer might involve applying phonological, morphological, or syntactic rules from spoken to sign language. This can sometimes hinder learning because of the modal and structural differences between sign and spoken languages. For deaf learners, native signers of a different sign language, transfer effects might facilitate learning through similarities in sign language structure and concepts.

Immersion in sign-language environments is one of the most effective modalities for learning sign language as a second language. Naturalistic exposure involves engaging with native signers in everyday contexts, allowing learners to observe and practice sign language through authentic communication. This method facilitates the acquisition of sign language vocabulary, grammar, and subtler aspects of sign language use, such as non-manual markers, facial expressions, and cultural nuances. Immersion experiences can range from living in deaf communities to participating in deaf events and gatherings, providing learners with invaluable opportunities to actively use the language and develop their signing skills in a supportive, naturalistic setting.

4.4 The Role of Family in the Sign Language Learning Process

The role of family in the sign language learning process is pivotal, exerting a profound influence on the developmental outcomes and linguistic competencies of deaf children. Family engagement in the learning process fosters a supportive environment for acquiring sign language and enhances the child's cognitive, emotional, and social development. This examination highlights the significance of familial involvement and its impact on educational outcomes and proposes strategies to encourage family engagement in sign language education.

Impact of Family Engagement on Learning Outcomes

(a) Linguistic Development: Families that actively learn and use sign language provide an essential foundation for deaf children's linguistic development. Early exposure to sign language within the family setting correlates with enhanced vocabulary acquisition, superior grammar understanding, and better communication skills. Studies have shown that deaf children of deaf parents who are exposed to sign language from birth often exhibit advanced linguistic abilities compared to their peers with hearing parents who do not sign.

(b) Cognitive Growth: Engagement with sign language at home fosters cognitive development. Sign language use stimulates brain areas involved in language processing and cognitive functions, promoting more robust neural pathways. Furthermore, bilingual exposure, such as sign and spoken or written language, enhances cognitive flexibility and problem-solving skills.

(c) Social-Emotional Benefits: Family involvement in sign language education supports the child's social-emotional development. It enables deaf children to communicate effectively with their family members, fostering a sense of belonging and self-esteem. This early, positive communication experience is crucial for developing secure attachment and emotional resilience.

Strategies for Involving Families in Sign Language Education

(a) Sign Language Workshops and Courses: Offering sign language workshops and courses tailored for families of deaf children can significantly boost their engagement. These programs should be accessible, preferably free or subsidized, and designed to accommodate families' schedules. Families can integrate signing into their daily routines by learning sign language together, making communication a shared journey.

(b) Online Resources and Learning Platforms: Leveraging online resources and learning platforms can provide families with flexible opportunities to learn sign language at their own pace. These resources can range from video tutorials and sign language apps to online courses, making it easier for families to access sign language education regardless of location.

(c) Family Involvement in Educational Settings: Encouraging family involvement in educational settings strengthens the link between home and school. Schools and educational programs can invite families to participate in sign language classes, workshops, and events, fostering a community of learners and enhancing the school's inclusive culture.

(d) Support Groups and Networks: Creating or facilitating access to support groups and networks for families can provide emotional support, resources, and motivation for learning sign language. These groups allow families to share experiences, challenges, and successes, creating a supportive community centered around sign language learning.

4.5 Interaction with Native Signers and the Deaf Community

Interaction with native signers is essential for acquiring proficiency in sign language. Engaging with the Deaf community allows learners to practice signing in real-life contexts, receive feedback, and learn cultural norms and etiquette associated with sign language use. This interaction facilitates language acquisition and fosters a deeper understanding and appreciation of deaf culture. Building relationships within the deaf community can be challenging for second language learners, who must navigate cultural differences and communication barriers. However, such engagement is invaluable in developing linguistic and cultural competence in sign languages. Encouraging respectful and meaningful participation in deaf communities is critical for successful sign language learning.

4.6 The Psychological Impact of Learning SL as a Second Language

Learning sign language as a second language can have profound psychological impacts on individuals, influencing their cognitive processes, social interactions, and identity formation. These effects extend beyond acquiring a new mode of communication and touching on aspects of personal growth, social empathy, and cultural integration.

Learning sign language can enhance cognitive flexibility, as it requires learners to engage with a linguistic system that differs significantly from spoken language in terms of modality and structure. This engagement demands and fosters adaptability in cognitive processing, potentially leading to improvements in problem-solving skills, creativity, and multitasking. Moreover, the visual-spatial nature of sign languages can enhance visual awareness and spatial reasoning skills that can be transferred to various cognitive tasks beyond language learning.

Acquiring sign language opens new cultural perspectives and insights. Learners often gain a deeper understanding of the deaf community, its values, and challenges. This increased cultural awareness can foster greater empathy and respect for diversity, encouraging learners to reassess their preconceived notions of deafness and disability. The process of cultural immersion and learning often leads to a broader appreciation of the complexity and richness of human communication, promoting a more inclusive viewpoint of societal diversity.

Sign language can improve overall communication skills, including nonverbal communication, which constitutes a significant portion of interpersonal interaction.

Learners become more attuned to the nuances of body language, facial expressions, and gestures, which improves their ability to understand and convey subtle cues during communication. This heightened sensitivity can enhance personal and professional relationships, making individuals more effective communicators in various contexts.

Learning sign language can also have therapeutic aspects, offering a new avenue for expression and understanding, which may be liberating for some individuals. The visual nature of sign languages provides a unique medium for self-expression, which can be particularly empowering for those who struggle with traditional verbal communication. Furthermore, learning and using a second language have been linked to increased self-efficacy and confidence and reduced anxiety in social situations.

The psychological impact of sign language learning is multifaceted. It influences cognitive abilities, social awareness, communication skills, identity, and emotional well-being. These effects highlight the profound influence of language learning on an individual's psychological landscape, underscoring the transformative power of embracing new languages and cultures.

4.7 Historical Perspectives on Sign Language Education

The historical development of sign language education is a rich tapestry of milestones, key figures, and evolving pedagogies that reflect broader societal attitudes towards deafness and communication diversity (Fig. 4.1). It began in the early eighteenth century and unfolded over centuries, marking a journey from marginalization to recognition and empowerment of the deaf community through education.

The formal teaching of sign language can be traced back to the early eighteenth century, with the establishment of the first public school for the deaf in Paris in 1755 by Charles-Michel de l'Épée. De l'Épée is often celebrated as a pioneering figure in deaf education for developing a method of instruction that incorporated sign language, a radical departure from the oralist approach that sought to teach deaf individuals to speak and lip-read. His work laid the foundation for what would become

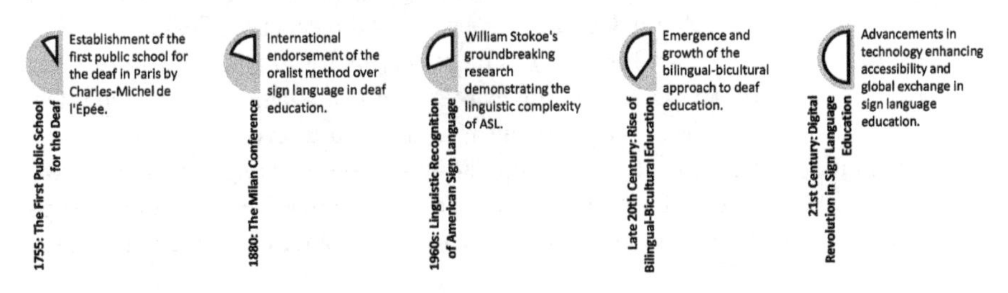

Fig. 4.1 Timeline of milestones in sign language education: tracing the evolution from marginalization to recognition and technological advancement

known as the "manual method" of deaf education, emphasizing the use of signs for instruction.

The historical trajectory of sign language education took a significant turn with the Milan Conference of 1880. This international gathering of deaf educators concluded with a strong endorsement of the oralist method, leading to widespread suppression of sign language in deaf education across many parts of the world. This period saw the rise of figures such as Alexander Graham Bell, who, despite his contributions to telecommunication, advocated for the oralist approach and eugenics policies affecting the deaf.

The twentieth century marked a revival and gradual recognition of sign languages and their educational value. William Stokoe, a linguist, played a crucial role in this transformation. In the 1960s, Stokoe's work at Gallaudet University challenged prevailing misconceptions by demonstrating that ASL possessed the full linguistic complexity of spoken languages. Recognizing ASL as a legitimate language ignited sign language education and research interest.

The latter half of the twentieth century saw a resurgence of bilingual-bicultural (Bi-Bi) approaches to deaf education, emphasizing the acquisition of both sign language and the dominant spoken/written language as essential to the cognitive and cultural development of deaf individuals. This period also witnessed the establishment and growth of deaf advocacy organizations that championed the rights of deaf individuals, including their right to education in sign language.

Digital technology has further transformed sign language education, making resources more accessible and facilitating the global exchange of educational methodologies and sign languages. Online platforms, social media, and mobile applications have played a significant role in spreading sign language literacy and empowering deaf learners.

4.8 Sign Language Education

Sign language education, whether aimed at deaf learners or those learning it as a second language, requires a nuanced approach that respects the visual-spatial nature of sign languages and the cultural context of deaf communities. Effective sign language education is built on several foundational principles designed to maximize learning outcomes and foster a deep understanding and respect for deaf culture.

Creating an immersive learning environment is crucial for sign language education. This approach involves surrounding learners with sign language through interaction with proficient signers, engagement in deaf cultural events, and using sign language in real-world contexts. Immersion allows learners to experience language as it is naturally used, thereby promoting fluency and comprehension. It also helps to understand nonverbal cues and the cultural nuances of sign language communication.

Given the visual nature of sign languages, effective educational strategies leverage visual learning tools and resources. These include videos, visual aids, flashcards, and other multimedia resources that facilitate learning sign vocabulary, grammar, and syntax. Visual tools help memorize signs and understand the conceptual and contextual use in communication.

Sign language cannot be separated from the culture of deaf communities. Thus, an integral sign language education principle is incorporating the deaf cultural context into the curriculum. This involves teaching about the history, values, norms, and practices of deaf communities. Engaging with the Deaf community and participating in its cultural and social events enriches the learning experience, providing learners with a deeper understanding and appreciation of the language and its cultural significance.

Sign language learners come from diverse backgrounds, varying exposures to sign languages, and differing learning needs. Thus, effective education employs differentiated instruction, tailoring teaching methods, and materials to meet the individual needs of learners. This can involve adjusting the pace of instruction, using various teaching strategies (e.g., visual and kinesthetic), and providing personalized feedback to support each student's unique learning journey.

Developing comprehensive language skills in sign language involves a multifaceted approach that addresses the unique aspects of sign language, including its visual-spatial nature, grammatical structures, and cultural nuances. Practical strategies for building language skills in sign language learners encompass the acquisition of vocabulary and grammar and the development of sociolinguistic competence. To facilitate this structured approach, educators can employ techniques such as

- Thematic Vocabulary Units: Grouping vocabulary into thematic units (e.g., family, food, and emotions) helps learners associate related signs and use them in context.
- Sequential Grammar Instruction: Introducing grammatical concepts in a logical sequence, starting with simple sentence structures and moving to more complex ones, supports gradual language acquisition.
- Visual Aids and Modeling: Visual aids and demonstration videos can help illustrate grammatical concepts and sign production techniques.

Sociolinguistic competence involves understanding the social and cultural contexts in which a language is used, including variations in registers, dialects, and etiquette. In sign language education, this means teaching learners how, when, and why signs and forms of expression are appropriate. Strategies to enhance sociolinguistic competence include the following.

- Exposure to Sign Language Variants: Introducing learners to regional variations and signing styles helps them appreciate the diversity within sign languages and prepares them for real-world interactions.
- Role-Playing and Social Situations: Simulating social interactions through role-playing can help learners practice appropriate sign language use in various contexts, from formal to casual settings.

- Cultural Immersion: Participation in Deaf community events and interactions with native signers provides invaluable experiences for understanding the cultural subtleties and social norms associated with sign language use.

Achieving fluency in sign language extends beyond vocabulary and grammar to include pragmatic skills and the ability to use language effectively in social situations. This involves understanding the nuances of conversation in sign languages, such as turn-taking cues, the role of eye gaze in establishing conversational roles, and the importance of facial expressions in conveying mood, tone, and grammatical information.

Educators can foster pragmatic competence through activities that mimic real-life interactions, allowing learners to practice storytelling, negotiate meaning, and engage in dialogue. Feedback from native signers and immersion in sign language environments are invaluable for developing these nuanced communication skills.

4.9 Comparative Analysis of SL Pedagogy Across Different Countries

The pedagogical practices in sign language education across various countries showcase a rich diversity influenced by cultural, historical, and societal factors. This analysis highlights the differences and similarities in approaches to sign language education, underlining the significant impact of cultural contexts on teaching methodologies, curriculum development, and educational outcomes for deaf learners.

United States: Bilingual-Bicultural Approach

Adopting the Bilingual-Bicultural (Bi-Bi) approach has been prominent in the United States. This methodology recognizes ASL as the primary language of deaf individuals, with English as the second language. The Bi-Bi approach emphasizes the importance of deaf culture and identity, integrating ASL and English instruction to promote linguistic competency and cultural understanding. The pedagogy is characterized by its emphasis on ASL proficiency as a foundation for learning, with English taught through various modalities, including reading and writing.

Sweden: Early Language Acquisition and Integration

Sweden is renowned for its early intervention and language acquisition programs for deaf children, where Swedish Sign Language (SSL) is introduced at a young age alongside Swedish. The Swedish education system emphasizes the integration of deaf and hard-of-hearing students into mainstream classrooms, supported by sign language interpreters and unique education resources. This inclusive approach reflects the societal value placed on equality and accessibility, aiming to provide deaf students with the skills necessary to navigate both deaf and hearing worlds.

Japan: Oralism and Sign Language Recognition

Japan's approach to deaf education has historically leaned towards oralism, focusing on teaching deaf children to speak and lip-read Japanese. However, recent decades have seen a gradual recognition and incorporation of Japanese Sign Language (JSL) into educational settings, following advocacy by the deaf community. The shift towards incorporating JSL signifies a growing acknowledgment of sign language as a legitimate linguistic and cultural form. However, challenges remain in fully integrating sign language pedagogy into the mainstream educational framework.

Ghana: Community-Based and Informal Learning

In Ghana and many parts of Africa, formal education for deaf individuals is limited by resources and accessibility. Consequently, sign language education often occurs within community settings and through informal learning channels. Ghanaian Sign Language (GSL) emerges from these community interactions, with education occurring in various non-traditional settings, including homes, social gatherings, and deaf clubs. This grassroots approach to sign language education underscores the importance of community and social networks in transmitting sign language and deaf culture.

Australia: Technology-Enhanced Learning

Australia's sign language education leverages technology to bridge geographical and accessibility gaps. Australian Sign Language (Auslan) education incorporates online learning platforms, video resources, and virtual classrooms to reach deaf students in remote areas. This use of technology reflects a broader trend towards digital inclusion and the democratization of education, allowing for greater flexibility and access to sign language learning resources.

Comparative Insights

While approaches to sign language pedagogy vary significantly across countries, commonalities emerge in recognizing sign languages as vital to deaf individuals' cultural and linguistic identity. The impact of cultural contexts on education is profound, influencing the acceptance, integration, and prioritization of sign language instruction. From the Bi-Bi approach in the United States to community-based learning in Ghana, each method reflects the underlying values and societal attitudes towards deafness and sign language. The gradual shift towards inclusive and technology-enhanced learning modalities worldwide suggests a promising direction for the future of sign language education, emphasizing the importance of accessibility, cultural respect, and linguistic rights.

4.10 The Role of Technology in Sign Language Education

In the evolving landscape of sign language education, technology is pivotal in transforming how learners access, engage with, and master sign language. Integrating technological tools from digital learning platforms into immersive virtual environments has opened new horizons for instruction, practice, and community engagement. Digital innovations enhance the learning experience, provide invaluable resources for training and exposure, and connect learners with the broader deaf community.

Digital learning platforms and applications are transformative tools that offer learners unparalleled access to resources, instructions, and community support. These digital avenues have democratized the learning of sign languages, making it possible for individuals around the globe to embark on their language learning journey, regardless of their proximity to physical classrooms or deaf communities. They allow learners to study sign language independently and according to their schedule. This flexibility is valuable for balancing learning with other commitments, such as work or family responsibilities. Moreover, these digital solutions often come with customizable learning paths, enabling learners to focus on areas of interest or challenges, thereby enhancing the efficiency and effectiveness of their study.

Many sign language apps and online platforms incorporate interactive elements such as quizzes, games, and practice exercises that enhance engagement and facilitate knowledge retention. These interactive features make learning more enjoyable and reinforce the acquisition of sign language vocabulary, grammar, and syntax through active participation and repetition.

In Fig. 4.2, TuniSigner and MemoSign are innovative applications designed to facilitate sign language learning, highlighting the growing intersection between technology and language education [22, 23]. TuniSigner focuses on providing a comprehensive learning experience for users interested in Tunisian Sign Language, offering an array of visual tools and interactive features to enhance engagement and

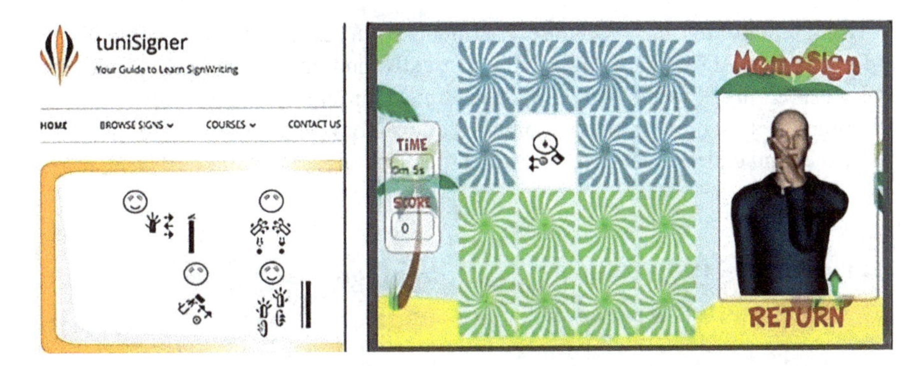

Fig. 4.2 TuniSigner and MemoSign applications to teach sign languages

retention using the SignWriting Notation System. On the other hand, MemoSign employs memory-based games and exercises to teach sign language, making the learning process fun and effective. Its design is centered on the cognitive processes involved in language acquisition, utilizing repetition and mnemonic devices to aid in memorizing and recalling sign language signs and phrases. The TuniSigner and MemoSign applications exemplify the innovative use of digital platforms in sign language education, providing learners with valuable resources that support a wide range of learning styles and objectives.

One more example of the use of technology in the classroom is introduced in the work of Yang et al., they developed an innovative concept in sign language translation and education through the development of Holographic Sign Language Interpreters [24]. This groundbreaking technology utilizes holograms to project three-dimensional sign language interpreters into any setting, providing a more immersive and interactive communication experience for deaf and hard-of-hearing individuals. Holographic interpreters can precisely mimic human movements, offering a dynamic and engaging way to learn and understand sign languages.

Given the visual nature of sign languages, digital platforms are uniquely suited for teaching. High-quality video demonstrations of signs and phrases allow learners to observe the minutiae of sign production, including hand shapes, movements, and facial expressions. Some platforms also offer slow-motion playback or angle changes to ensure that learners fully grasp each sign. Additionally, multimedia resources can include cultural notes, stories from the deaf community, and interviews with native signers, providing context and depth to the language learning experience.

One of the most significant advantages of digital learning platforms and apps is their ability to connect learners to a broader community. Many apps integrate social features, allowing users to interact, share their progress, and practice with others. This sense of community motivates learners and exposes them to various signing styles and dialects, enriching their learning experiences. Furthermore, feedback from the community or instructors within these platforms can offer valuable corrections and insights, facilitating improvement and confidence in sign-language skills.

Digital platforms and apps are continuously updated with new content that reflects changes in language use, cultural trends, and educational methodologies. This ensured that learners had access to the most current and relevant materials. In addition, the scalability of digital solutions allows for the inclusion of multiple sign languages and dialects, catering to a broad spectrum of learners' interests and needs.

4.11 Future Directions in Sign Language Education Research

Sign language education research landscape is dynamic, reflecting the evolving understanding of linguistic diversity, technological advancements, and educational methodologies. Exploring future directions in this field involves identifying gaps in knowledge, recognizing emerging trends, and pinpointing potential areas of study. These efforts are crucial for enhancing the efficacy of sign language education and ensuring it meets the diverse needs of learners. This exploration offers a roadmap for future research projects to advance sign language education (Fig. 4.3).

4.12 Conclusion

As detailed in this chapter, the exploration of sign language acquisition and education traverses the multifaceted dimensions of how individuals learn and internalize sign languages within various contexts and educational frameworks. Through an exhaustive analysis, the chapter illuminates the inherent complexity of sign

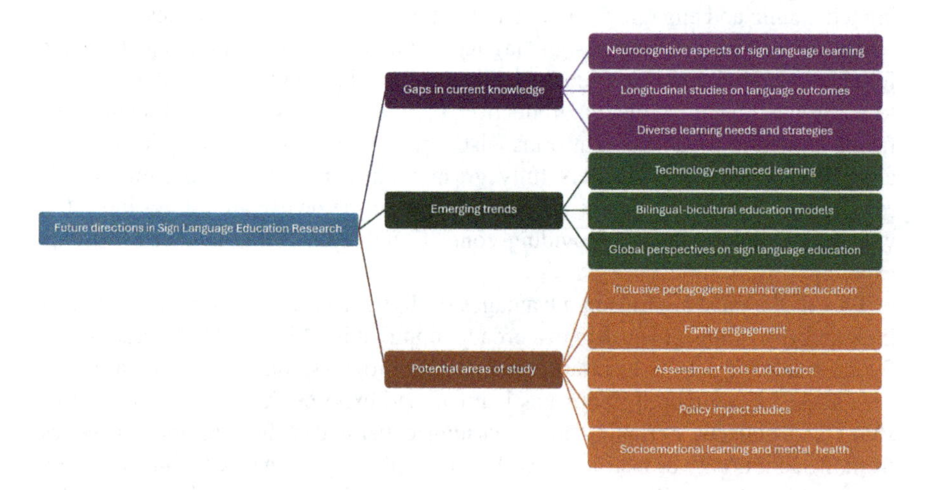

Fig. 4.3 Trends and future directions in sign language education

language learning, underscored by the diverse methodologies that cater to acquiring these languages as either a first or subsequent mode of communication. The discourse extends beyond mere acquisition, delving into the pedagogical underpinnings that guide educational practices and the technological innovations reshaping the landscape of sign language education.

The historical development of sign language education, the theoretical and practical challenges of first and second language acquisition, the pivotal role of family involvement, and the transformative power of technology culminate in a comprehensive understanding of this field's current state and prospects. This examination highlights the universal and unique aspects of language learning mechanisms and the societal, cultural, and technological dynamics influencing the education of deaf individuals and sign language learners worldwide.

The comparative analysis of sign language pedagogy across different countries reveals a tapestry of educational practices shaped by cultural and societal values that reflect a global movement towards recognizing and embracing the linguistic rights and cultural identity of deaf communities. Furthermore, the discussion on future research directions opens avenues for addressing gaps in our understanding, leveraging technological advancements, and fostering inclusive educational practices that accommodate the diverse needs of learners.

In conclusion, sign language acquisition and education stand at a crossroads of linguistic research, educational theory, and technological innovation. The insights garnered from this chapter underscore the necessity for continued exploration, advocacy, and policy-making that support the growth and development of sign language education. By embracing the complexity and diversity of sign languages, educators, researchers, and policymakers can enrich the educational experiences of deaf learners, ensuring their full participation in a linguistically diverse world. The journey through sign language education is not only about overcoming barriers but also about celebrating the rich cultural heritage and linguistic identity of the deaf community, paving the way for a more inclusive and understanding society.

Quiz Time

1. What does the first language acquisition process in deaf children primarily rely on?

(A) Auditory-oral modality
(B) Visual-spatial modality
(C) Kinesthetic learning

2. What concept supports the idea that there is an optimal period for language acquisition in early life?

(A) Cognitive flexibility theory
(B) Critical period hypothesis
(C) Universal Grammar

3. According to the chapter, which hemisphere of the brain primarily controls sign language?

(A) Right hemisphere
(B) Left hemisphere
(C) Both hemispheres equally

4. What type of activities are cited as improving ASL phonological awareness in deaf children?

(A) Rhyme, rhythm, and handshape awareness activities
(B) Syntax and grammar exercises
(C) Reading and writing practice

5. What is highlighted as a consequence of delayed exposure to sign language in deaf children born to hearing parents?

(A) Improved adaptability to multiple languages
(B) Enhanced cognitive skills
(C) Linguistic, cognitive, and social repercussions

6. Which approach to sign language education emphasizes the acquisition of both sign language and the dominant spoken/written language?

(A) Bilingual-Bicultural (Bi-Bi) approach
(B) Total Communication
(C) Oralism

7. What does immersion in a sign-language environment primarily facilitate?

(A) Social isolation
(B) Quick mastery of foreign languages
(C) Naturalistic language acquisition and fluency

8. What role do 'non-manual markers' play in sign languages as discussed in the chapter?

(A) They are rarely used and unimportant
(B) They convey grammatical information like questions or exclamations
(C) They only indicate the signer's emotions

9. Which method is NOT mentioned as a way to involve families in sign language education?

(A) Offering sign language workshops and courses
(B) Encouraging families to develop their own sign language
(C) Leveraging online resources and learning platforms

10. What significant impact does early exposure to sign language have on deaf children?

(A) It delays their language development

(B) It significantly improves their language development
(C) It has no noticeable impact

References

1. Hall, M.L., Hall, W.C., Caselli, N.K.: Deaf children need language, not (just) speech. First Language. 39, 367–395 (2019). https://doi.org/10.1177/0142723719834102.
2. Sandler, W., Lillo-Martin, D.: Natural Sign Languages. In: Aronoff, M. and Ress-Miller, J. (eds.) The Handbook of Linguistics. pp. 533–562. Wiley (2003). https://doi.org/10.1002/9780470756409.ch22.
3. Bellugi, U., Poizner, H., Klima, E.S.: Language, modality and the brain. Trends in Neurosciences. 12, 380–388 (1989). https://doi.org/10.1016/0166-2236(89)90076-3.
4. Della Chiesa, B., Scott, J., Hinton, C. eds: Neuroscientific research and the study of sign language. In: Languages in a Global World. pp. 181–197. OECD (2012). https://doi.org/10.1787/9789264123557-16-en.
5. Wilbur, R.B.: What does the study of signed languages tell us about 'language'? SL&L. 9, 5–32 (2006). https://doi.org/10.1075/sll.9.1.04wil.
6. Garcia, B., Sallandre, M.-A.: Transcription systems for sign languages: A sketch of the different graphical representations of sign language and their characteristics. In: Müller, C., Cienki, A., Fricke, E., Ladewig, S., McNeill, D., and Tessendorf, S. (eds.) Handbücher zur Sprach- und Kommunikationswissenschaft / Handbooks of Linguistics and Communication Science (HSK) 38/1. pp. 1125–1140. DE GRUYTER (2013). https://doi.org/10.1515/9783110261318.1125.
7. Hurford, J.R.: The evolution of the critical period for language acquisition. Cognition. 40, 159–201 (1991). https://doi.org/10.1016/0010-0277(91)90024-X.
8. Ruben, R.J.: A Time Frame of Critical/Sensitive Periods of Language Development. Acta Oto-Laryngologica. 117, 202–205 (1997). https://doi.org/10.3109/00016489709117769.
9. Capirci, O., Iverson, J.M., Montanari, S., Volterra, V.: Gestural, signed and spoken modalities in early language development: The role of linguistic input. Bilingualism. 5, (2002). https://doi.org/10.1017/S1366728902000123.
10. Holcomb, L., Golos, D., Moses, A., Broadrick, A.: Enriching Deaf Children's American Sign Language Phonological Awareness: A Quasi-Experimental Study. The Journal of Deaf Studies and Deaf Education. 27, 26–36 (2021). https://doi.org/10.1093/deafed/enab028.
11. Lieberman, A.M.: Attention-getting skills of deaf children using American Sign Language in a preschool classroom. Applied Psycholinguistics. 36, 855–873 (2015). https://doi.org/10.1017/S0142716413000532.
12. Toth, A.: Bridge of Signs: Can Sign Language Empower Non-Deaf Children to Triumph over Their Communication Disabilities? aad. 154, 85–95 (2009). https://doi.org/10.1353/aad.0.0084.
13. Le Roux, A., Stander, M.: Early language intervention in deaf children of hearing parents. PLING. 37, 15–27 (2021). https://doi.org/10.5785/37-1-974.
14. Bernhardt, E.B., Krashen, S.D.: Second Language Acquisition and Second Language Learning. The Modern Language Journal. 73, 483 (1989). https://doi.org/10.2307/326882.
15. Spolsky, B.: Attitudinal aspects of second language learning. Language Learning. 19, 271–275 (1969). https://doi.org/10.1111/j.1467-1770.1969.tb00468.x.
16. Benati, A.G., Angelovska, T.: Second Language Acquisition: A theoretical introduction to real-world applications. Bloomsbury Academic (2016). https://doi.org/10.5040/9781474298414.
17. Meisel, J.M.: First and second language acquisition: parallels and differences. Cambridge Univ. Press, Cambridge (2013).
18. Schönström, K.: Sign languages and second language acquisition research: An introduction. Journal of the European Second Language Association. 5, 30–43 (2021). 10.22599/jesla.73.

19. Mayer, C.: Issues in second language literacy education with learners who are deaf. International Journal of Bilingual Education and Bilingualism. 12, 325–334 (2009). https://doi.org/10.1080/13670050802153368.
20. Hoiting, N., Slobin, D.I.: 4 From Gestures to Signs in the Acquisition of Sign Language. In: Duncan, S.D., Cassell, J., and Levy, E.T. (eds.) Gesture Studies. pp. 51–65. John Benjamins Publishing Company, Amsterdam (2007). https://doi.org/10.1075/gs.1.06hoi.
21. Woll, B.: Second Language Acquisition of Sign Language. In: Chapelle, C.A. (ed.) The Encyclopedia of Applied Linguistics. Wiley (2012). https://doi.org/10.1002/9781405198431.wbeal1050.
22. Bouzid, Y., Jemni, M.: tuniSigner: A Virtual Interpreter to Learn Sign Writing. In: 2014 IEEE 14th International Conference on Advanced Learning Technologies. pp. 601–605. IEEE, Athens, Greece (2014). https://doi.org/10.1109/ICALT.2014.176.
23. Bouzid, Y., Khenissi, M.A., Jemni, M.: Designing a game generator as an educational technology for the deaf learners. In: 2015 5th International Conference on Information & Communication Technology and Accessibility (ICTA). pp. 1–6. IEEE (2015).
24. Yang, F., Mousas, C., Adamo, N.: Holographic sign language avatar interpreter: A user interaction study in a mixed reality classroom. Computer Animation & Virtual. 33, e2082 (2022). https://doi.org/10.1002/cav.2082.

Chapter 5
Sign Language Processing Tasks

5.1 Introduction

Natural Language Processing (NLP) primarily deals with spoken and written languages, focusing on text and speech data. In NLP, different techniques are developed to handle tasks such as part-of-speech tagging, syntactic parsing, semantic role annotation, sentiment analysis, machine translation, etc. These tasks are generally performed on linear, sequential data, following specific rules and conventions standard across most spoken languages. In contrast, Sign Language Processing (SLP) focuses on visual-spatial languages, which involve using hand gestures, facial expressions, and body movements to convey meaning, as explained in previous chapters. Sign languages are characterized by their simultaneous structure, where multiple elements can be expressed simultaneously, and their reliance on spatial and temporal information.

The SLP occupies a contested space within the broader scope of Artificial Intelligence and computer vision [1]. Some argue for its inclusion within Natural Language Processing (NLP) due to shared language understanding and generation objectives [2]. The intersection of SLP and NLP presents a unique opportunity to expand the capabilities of computational linguistics to be more inclusive and representative of the diversity of human languages, as shown in Fig. 5.1. This entails addressing the technical challenges and fostering collaboration between computer scientists, linguists, and the sign language community to develop socially impactful and scientifically robust solutions. Proponents of separation highlight the fundamental differences between spoken and signed languages, emphasizing the visual modality of sign languages and the unique role of facial expressions and body language in conveying meaning [1]. This debate reflects the ongoing discussion around the nature of language itself and the boundaries between spoken and signed modalities. Further research is needed to determine the optimal placement for SLP, considering the potential benefits of cross-pollination between NLP and computer

A. Othman, *Sign Language Processing*,
https://doi.org/10.1007/978-3-031-68763-1_5

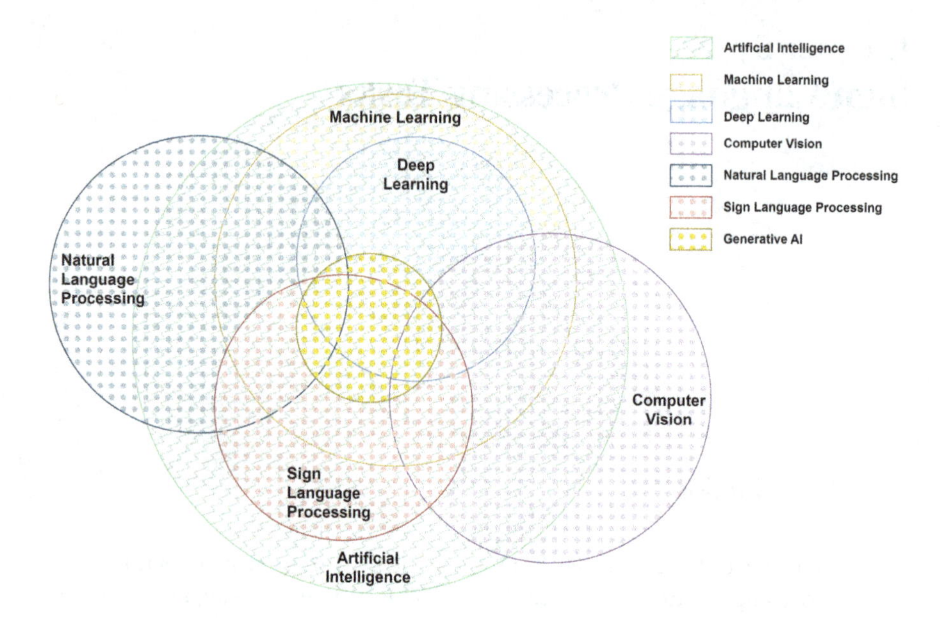

Fig. 5.1 Venn diagram showing the intersections of Artificial Intelligence, Machine Learning, Deep Learning, Computer Vision, Natural Language Processing, Sign Language Processing, and Generative AI

vision techniques while acknowledging the distinct linguistic features of signed languages.

Sign language processing encompasses a range of techniques and tools for analyzing and recognizing sign language. In [3, 4], authors highlighted this field's importance in developing interactive educational tools and integrating deaf-mute individuals into mainstream society. Carreiras emphasizes the cognitive mechanisms involved in sign language comprehension and production, focusing on the effects of age of acquisition and iconicity [5]. [6] introduces the SignWriting system, a practical writing system for deaf sign languages, and its application in SLP. These studies collectively underscore the significance of sign language processing in facilitating communication and understanding for the deaf and mute community. Othman et al. presented a statistical machine translation from written text to American Sign Language annotated in Gloss format [7].

As a result, SLP necessitates specialized methods to address the unique difficulties presented by sign languages, such as generating the desired outcome using NLP techniques and adhering strictly to its spelling, specific terminology, and phrases. From the literature, Fig. 5.2 illustrates the main tasks of SLP commonly discussed in the research. All tasks will be discussed in detail in the current chapter.

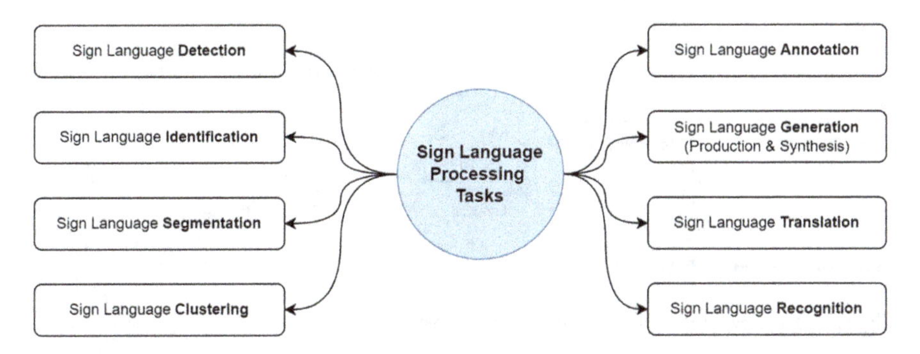

Fig. 5.2 Sign language processing tasks

5.2 Sign Language Detection

Sign language detection is a subtask within Sign Language Processing (SLP) that focuses on identifying the presence of sign language in a visual input (like a video stream or image) [8]. It is an initial step before more complex processing, like sign recognition or translation, can occur. The task has seen significant advancements in recent years. Patil et al. introduced a system using sensor gloves to capture American Sign Language (ASL) and translate it to English [9], while Titarmare et al. highlighted the role of computer vision and artificial intelligence in recognizing and interpreting sign language gestures [9]. Iyer et al. proposed a model for real-time sign language detection using action recognition [10]. Mondhe et al. developed a mobile application, SignDetect, that recognizes sign language, translates it to English, and generates text and audio formats [11]. These studies collectively underscore the potential of technology in bridging communication gaps for individuals with hearing impairments.

Definition Sign Language Detection is a computational task that involves identifying instances of sign language use within video content. This process distinguishes segments containing sign language from those that do not, without interpreting the meaning of the signs.

As shown in Fig. 5.3, the process begins with an image or video input. This input is first subjected to a '*Sign Language Detection Task*,' which is pivotal in determining whether the content contains sign language. The detection task acts as a filter: if the input is recognized as sign language, the process moves forward to the next stage; if not, the input is dismissed as '*Not Sign Language*,' and the process halts for that input. After successful sign language detection, the flowchart proceeds to the 'Sign Language Classification' stage. Here, the identified sign language is further analyzed to classify it into one of several specific sign languages. The examples in the chart include American Sign Language, British Sign Language, or any other sign language not explicitly listed. This classification is considered for subsequent tasks, such as translation or interpretation, as each sign language has its unique lexicon and grammatical structure.

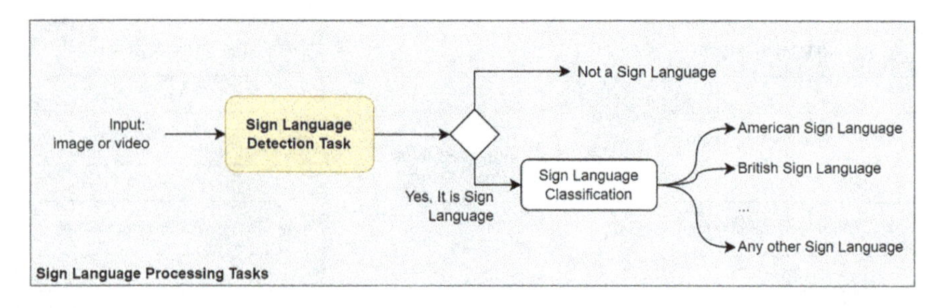

Fig. 5.3 Overview of the sign language detection task

Sign Language Detection entails identifying the presence of sign language within an image or video input. It is complicated by the intricate nature of sign language, which involves various factors such as hand shapes, positions, movements, facial expressions, and body postures. Computer vision and machine learning techniques are commonly used to tackle this challenge, encompassing the following subsections.

Skin Color Detection (SCD)

Many studies have explored SCD in sign language recognition and detection tasks. Kawulok and Konwar et al. developed systems for sign language detection using the SCD technique, with the former achieving higher effectiveness than general skin detection models [12, 13]. Khan et al. further enhanced this approach by incorporating heuristic rules and an Artificial Neural Network for SCD, achieving real-time translation of ASL [14]. In [15], authors utilized SCD in a sign language recognition system, achieving a high average recognition rate. These studies collectively demonstrate the potential of SCD in sign language recognition systems.

SCD primarily focuses on identifying the nuances of sign language gestures through the analysis of skin color segmentation. By utilizing advanced algorithms, the system detects human skin regions in video or real-time camera feeds, isolating the hands and fingers, which are pivotal in sign language communication. This method enhances gesture recognition accuracy by minimizing background noise and focusing on the essential components of sign language. Examples of techniques used in SCD tasks are illustrated in Fig. 5.4 and described as follow:

- **Motion Detection**: Since sign language involves movement, algorithms that detect and track motion can help identify signing activity. Optical flow or background subtraction detects dynamic regions in video frames.
- **Hand Shape Recognition**: Advanced pattern recognition techniques are applied to identify hand configurations, which are fundamental in differentiating signs. This can involve deep learning models trained to classify hand shapes.

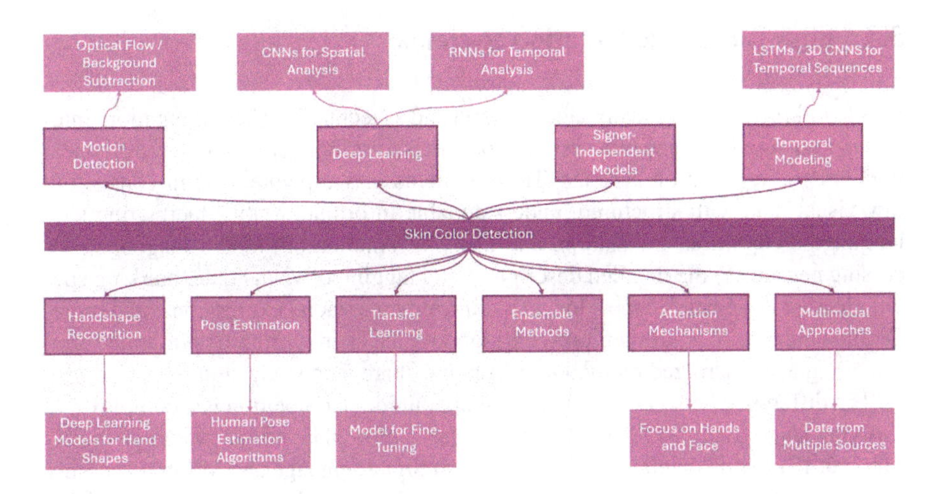

Fig. 5.4 Skin color detection techniques

- **Pose Estimation**: Human pose estimation algorithms detect the position and orientation of the head, body, and arms, which are critical for understanding the context of the used signs.
- **Deep Learning**: Convolutional Neural Networks (CNNs) and Recurrent Neural Networks (RNNs) are handy for processing sign language's spatial and temporal aspects, respectively. They can analyze sequences of images (frames) to detect sign language patterns over time.
- **Transfer Learning**: To handle the scarcity of labeled sign language datasets, transfer learning techniques are often used where a model pre-trained on a large dataset is fine-tuned on a smaller sign language dataset.
- **Temporal Modeling**: Techniques like Long Short-Term Memory Networks (LSTMs) or 3D CNNs can model temporal sequences to differentiate between signing and non-signing activities over a period.
- **Ensemble Methods**: Combining the predictions from multiple models or feature detectors can improve the reliability of sign language detection.
- **Attention Mechanisms**: These focus the model on the most relevant parts of the video frames, such as the signer's hands and face, to improve detection accuracy.
- **Signer-Independent Models**: These are designed to generalize across signers with varying styles and speeds of signing and different physical appearances.
- **Multimodal Approaches**: Incorporating data from multiple sources, such as depth sensors or wearable devices, can provide additional information to improve detection accuracy.

5.3 Sign Language Notation Systems

Before talking about sign language notation and ss technology becoming more integrated into sign language processing, it becomes ever more crucial to have practical notation and convention systems. These systems play a pivotal role in connecting raw visual data with structured, understandable information, thus facilitating sign language recognition, translation, and analysis. Annotation in sign language processing pertains to the detailed description and tagging of visual data, marking specific features like handshapes, locations, movements, facial expressions, and more. On the other hand, notation represents sign languages in written or symbolic form, providing a standardized method to document, share, and study signs.

The difference between sign language annotation and notation is a complex and evolving study area. Dhanjal et al. and Miller explore the various systems of notation [16, 17], with Dhanjal focusing on Indian Sign Language and Miller discussing the development of notational conventions. Koizumi et al. and Dubot et al. delve into the challenges and potential solutions for annotating sign language [18, 19]. Koizumi addresses the grammatical analysis of Japanese sign language and Dubot proposes a formalism for parsing sign language. In [20, 21], researchers highlighted the need for automation and standardization in the annotation process, with Chaaban presenting a semi-automatic annotation system and Crasborn discussing the need for unified annotation standards. Lastly, Sallandre critiques existing notation systems questioning the use of gloss-based notations and comparing different notation system [22].

Definition Sign Language Notation refers to the set of systems designed to transcribe sign languages into a written or graphical form. This includes various methods for capturing the complex movements and gestures of sign language in a two-dimensional medium for the purposes of analysis, learning, and preservation.

Many studies have explored sign language annotation and notation, focusing on manual and non-manual features. Aitpayev et al. and Dreuw et al. have developed tools for semi-automatic annotation [23, 24], with Aitpayev using depth and RGB cameras and Dreuw creating an interface for the ELAN software. Othman et al. and Chételat-Pelé et al. have proposed annotation systems [25, 26], with Othman introducing an XML-gloss system and Chételat-Pelé focusing on non-manual gestures. Studies from [21, 27] have emphasized the need for standardized annotation practices, with Schembri discussing the properties of such standards and creating joint annotation guidelines for glossing sign language corpora. Koizumi et al. applied these practices to specific sign languages on annotating a Japanese sign language [18]. Braffort et al. developed a new annotation software for French sign language videos [28].

Several sign language annotation and notation systems have gained prominence over the years, each bringing its unique approach and strengths:

Stokoe Notation

The Stokoe Notation System, developed by Dr. William Stokoe in the 1960s, represents a seminal advancement in sign language linguistics and remains a cornerstone in the study and transcription of sign languages. Stokoe's work was groundbreaking because it was among the first to challenge the prevailing belief that sign languages were mere gestures rather than languages with their grammar and syntax [29]. Stokoe's system introduced a descriptive framework to analyze the components of signs in ASL, focusing on three primary aspects: tabula, designator, and signation. These correspond to the location of the sign, the handshape, and the movement, respectively, and collectively form what is known as cheremes (from Greek 'cheir', meaning 'hand').

His seminal work, "*Sign Language Structure: An Outline of the Visual Communication Systems of the American Deaf*" [29], provided the foundation for sign language to be recognized as a natural language with its syntax and morphology. The Stokoe Notation System was utilized in this study to systematically describe the phonemic units of ASL, paving the way for further research and acceptance of sign languages globally.

Stokoe's contributions transcended linguistic boundaries and had a profound sociocultural impact, as they played a pivotal role in the Deaf community's fight for recognition of their language and, by extension, their culture. The Stokoe Notation System is not without its limitations, however, and has since been supplemented by other systems that aim to capture the multidimensional and dynamic nature of sign language, such as SignWriting and the Hamburg Sign Language Notation System (HamNoSys), which allow for a more comprehensive representation of the spatial and kinetic aspects of sign languages [30].

Despite its limitations, the Stokoe Notation System remains a fundamental reference point in sign language research and documentation, serving as a testament to Stokoe's legacy in linguistics and the ongoing effort to understand and preserve the linguistic diversity of human language.

Hamburg Notation System

The Hamburg Notation System (HamNoSys)[1] stands as a pioneering and comprehensive symbolic system explicitly designed for the notation of sign languages. Developed at the University of Hamburg, HamNoSys transcends linguistic boundaries, offering a universal platform for documenting the intricate details of sign language gestures. Unlike conventional writing systems that rely heavily on the representation of spoken languages, HamNoSys is meticulously structured to capture the visual-spatial nature of sign language, including hand shapes, orientations,

[1] Learn more about HamNoSys: https://web.dgs-korpus.de/hamnosys-97.html

movements, facial expressions, and body postures. Its versatility and precision make it an invaluable tool for researchers, educators, and technologists, enabling the detailed analysis, preservation, and sharing of sign languages across different cultures and regions.

HamNoSys is a complex but valuable tool for SLP [31]. It has been used in various applications, including the transcription of children's signing [32], the development of an open-source parser for multilingual sign language encoding [33], and the creation of an interactive notation editor for signed speech annotation [34]. HamNoSys has also been applied to continuous sign language recognition, significantly reducing Word Error Rate [35]. Furthermore, it has been used to develop a system for converting HamNoSys to SiGML for sign language automation [36].

SignWriting

SignWriting[2] is a different writing system that brings sign language's dynamic and visually oriented nature to the page. Developed by Valerie Sutton in the 1970s, provides a graphical representation of sign languages, capturing the movement, facial expressions, and specific hand shapes that constitute the essence of signed communication. Unlike other notation systems designed primarily for research, SignWriting is accessible to deaf and hearing individuals. It is a practical tool for everyday use, education, and literary creation within the deaf community. Its intuitive design allows for the recording and dissemination of sign languages in a visually analogous manner, fostering literacy and promoting a deeper understanding of the linguistic complexities of sign languages.

The SignWriting notation system has been widely recognized for its practicality and effectiveness in representing sign languages [6, 37]. It has been applied to various sign languages, including Japanese Sign Language (JSL) [38]. Efforts have been made to incorporate SignWriting into information technology, such as developing a recognition system [39] and an avatar-based system for interpreting SignWriting notations [40]. The system has also been used in the computer processing of deaf sign languages, enabling various language and document processing tasks [6]. However, the system has been criticized for its complexity and the time required to compose signs [38]. Despite these challenges, SignWriting remains a valuable tool for representing sign languages.

[2] Learn more about SignWriting: https://www.signwriting.org/

Gloss Notation Convention

Gloss notation, in the context of sign language research and documentation, is not a notation system in the same way that systems like Stokoe Notation or SignWriting are. Instead, it is a method to transcribe sign languages into written form, primarily through words or abbreviations from a spoken language (often English for ASL) to represent signs. Each gloss typically corresponds to a single sign and is written in capital letters to distinguish it from the surrounding text in a sentence.

While glossing is common for annotating sign language data, especially in academic research, it must provide a detailed phonetic or phonological representation of signs. Instead, it is a convenient shorthand to document sign language's lexical or semantic aspects, often used with video recordings for clarity. Gloss notation is more about providing a readable, straightforward transcription than capturing the full range of motion, expression, and spatial features inherent in sign language communication.

Although gloss notation doesn't capture the nuanced physical movements, facial expressions, and spatial orientations integral to sign languages, it provides a succinct and accessible means to document and analyze the lexical and semantic components of sign language utterances. This method is invaluable for researchers, educators, and students, facilitating the study of sign language structure, development of learning materials, and cross-linguistic comparisons. Gloss notation, while not exhaustive in its representation of sign languages, plays a critical role in the broader efforts to understand and disseminate the rich linguistic intricacies of signed languages.

Many studies have explored the development and application of gloss notation conventions in sign language. Ormel et al. investigate the formulation of uniform gloss notation practices for sign language corpora [41], underscoring the necessity of standardization in linguistic documentation. Mesch et al. further contribute to this discussion with a specific focus on creating gloss annotations within the context of Swedish Sign Language [42], adding a cross-linguistic perspective to the conversation. Pizzuto et al. interrogate the methodological and theoretical considerations inherent in employing gloss-based notations [43], particularly when analyzing signed texts, suggesting a complex interplay between notation systems and linguistic interpretation. For the Arabic language, Aouiti et al. introduced a specialized system tailored for Arabic Sign Language [44, 45], designed to navigate the perceived absence of fixed rules and grammatical frameworks in sign language. In advancing the discourse, Hanke et al. present a gloss-based scripting language to enhance the transcription and study of sign languages [46].

Developing and implementing gloss notation conventions in sign language studies have been pivotal in advancing linguistic research. However, as these diverse studies demonstrate, achieving standardization remains a challenging yet critical effort to ensure accurate representation and analysis of signed languages.

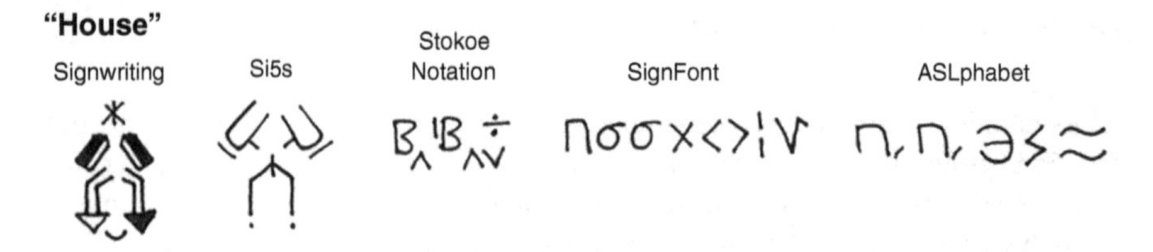

Fig. 5.5 Comparison of some ASL writing systems (Source: Wikipedia (Si5s Notation Comparison: https://en.wikipedia.org/wiki/Si5s))

Other Sign Language Notation System

Other sign language notation systems were developed. The Si5s system, the ASLphabet, SignFont, the Sign Language Notation System (SLNS), Prosodic Sign Language Notation (ProSign), and Typannot represent significant efforts in this domain (Fig. 5.5).

The Si5s notation system[3] is a writing system for ASL that Robert Arnold Augustus developed to faithfully represent the physical components of signs using a set of graphical symbols. It captures the intricacies of handshapes, orientations, locations, movements, and facial expressions, presenting them in a linear, sequential format. Unlike other notation systems, Si5s was designed to be an easily learnable and writable system for the everyday communication of ASL users.

ASLphabet,[4] another notational approach, was created as a simplified tool primarily for educational purposes. Its focus is on ease of use, targeting new learners of ASL, especially young children and their families (Bahan, 2008). ASLphabet aims to be intuitive, using letters and numbers associated with handshapes and simple illustrations to denote movement and facial expressions.

5.4 Sign Language Annotation

Moving from the notation systems' specificities, we now explore the rich landscape of annotation systems for sign language. While notation systems provide a structured method for representing the physical aspects of sign language, annotation systems aim to capture, organize, and elucidate the functional, contextual, and semantic information of signed data. These systems are designed to interface with sign language corpora, enabling researchers to align the sign language data with its corresponding annotations for a more nuanced analysis. This allows the documentation of the signs and their multifaceted uses and meanings within natural discourse. The following section will delve into the methodologies, technologies, and frameworks that underpin annotation systems for sign language, laying the groundwork

[3] Learn more about Si5s notation: https://dbpedia.org/page/Si5s

[4] Learn more about ASLphabet: http://www.asl-phabet.com/

for a comprehensive understanding of how these systems contribute to the study and dissemination of sign languages.

Definition Sign Language Annotation is the process of adding descriptive information to sign language data, typically video, to label specific signs, expressions, and non-manual features. This can include details on hand shapes, movements, facial expressions, and body language, which are critical for understanding and analyzing sign language.

Sign Language Phonetic Annotator-Analyzer

The Sign Language Phonetic Annotator-Analyzer is a detailed annotation framework designed to capture the phonetic and phonological nuances of sign languages comprehensively [47]. Unlike broader transcription systems focusing on signs' lexical or semantic aspects, the tool aims to document sign production's intricate physical and visual components, including handshapes, movements, locations, orientations, and non-manual features such as facial expressions and body posture. This level of detail makes SLPAS a tool for linguists and researchers dedicated to exploring the depth of sign language phonetics and phonology, offering insights into the subtle variations and patterns that characterize sign language structure and use.

ELAN

ELAN[5] is a tool for creating annotations on video and audio resources. Developed by the Max Planck Institute for Psycholinguistics in Nijmegen, the Netherlands, ELAN is specifically designed to analyze and document sign languages and other linguistic and non-linguistic data. It allows researchers to annotate media files with multiple layers of information, including but not limited to gestures, sign language, spoken language transcription, and paralinguistic features. While it can work with data annotated in various sign language notation systems, ELAN is a software tool for annotation rather than a notation system.

ELAN's capability to accommodate a range of annotation types—from broad phonetic transcriptions to fine-grained phonological descriptions—makes it an invaluable resource for documenting, analyzing, and preserving sign languages. Its use has become widespread in the linguistic community, facilitating the creation of comprehensive sign language corpora and enhancing collaborative efforts between researchers and the Deaf community [41].

[5] About ELAN: https://archive.mpi.nl/tla/elan

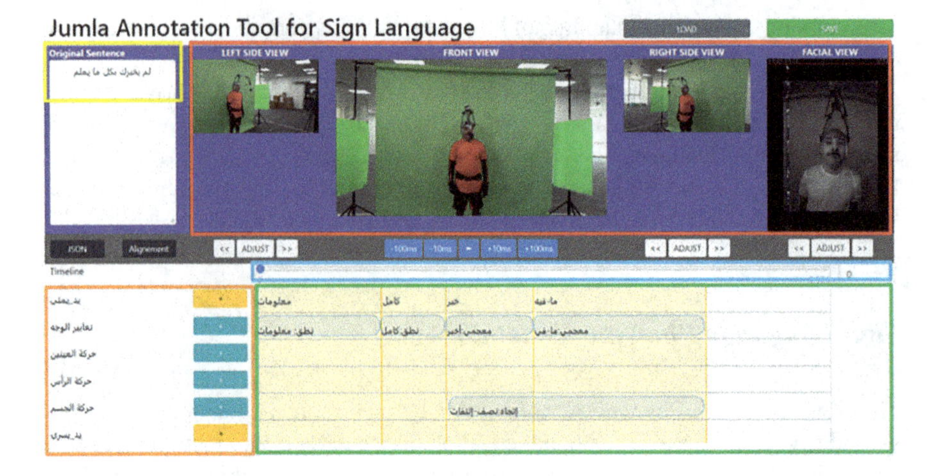

Fig. 5.6 Jumla annotation tool for sign language user interface

JUMLA Sign Language Annotation Tool

The development of the Jumla Annotation Tool for Sign Language[6] is a significant advancement in sign language processing. Othman et al. discussed the tool's use in annotating the Jumla Qatari Sign Language Corpus, focusing on Arabic glosses and managing video records [48]. In 2023, Elghoul et al. further expands on this, presenting the JUMLA-QSL-22 corpus and the tool's role in its creation [49]. These studies highlight the tool's potential to facilitate the development of computational sign language tools. The Jumla Annotation Tool shares similarities with other sign language annotation tools, such as the SLAN tool [50] and the Sign Language Phonetic Annotator-Analyzer [47], in its focus on video annotation and the creation of sign language corpora. However, the Jumla Annotation Tool's specific features and functionalities, particularly in Qatari Sign Language, set it apart from these other tools (Fig. 5.6).

5.5 Conclusion

This chapter provided an in-depth analysis of Sign Language Processing (SLP) and its position within the broader domains of Natural Language Processing (NLP), computer vision, and Artificial Intelligence (AI). The chapter delineated the specialized methodologies necessitated by the unique characteristics of sign languages and

[6] Jumla Annotation Tool for Sign Language: https://github.com/madainnovation/Jumla-Sign-Language-Annotation-Tool-By-Mada-Center

discussed the technical aspects and advancements in sign language detection, recognition, and translation. The application of various computational techniques such as Skin Color Detection (SCD), motion and pose estimation, and the adaptation of deep learning algorithms were critically examined for their roles in the evolution of SLP.

Furthermore, the chapter evaluated the significance of different sign language notation systems, including the Stokoe Notation, Hamburg Notation System (HamNoSys), and SignWriting, emphasizing their contributions to the transcription and documentation of sign languages. These systems' implications for computational applications were also considered, showcasing their importance in facilitating communication for the Deaf and hard-of-hearing individuals.

The subsequent chapter will continue the exploration of the advanced tasks in SLP by examining advanced computational models and their practical applications. This chapter will focus on the specifics of real-time sign language translation systems, the development of SLP-based educational tools, and the implications of these technologies for the Deaf community. It will provide a detailed exposition of the current state of research in sign language annotation and discuss the challenges and prospects for future developments in SLP.

Quiz Time

1. What is Sign Language Processing primarily concerned with?

(A) Developing methods for text-to-speech conversion
(B) Handling visual-spatial languages using hand gestures and facial expressions
(C) Improving audio recognition algorithms

2. Which area does SLP overlap with according to the document?

(A) Only Natural Language Processing
(B) Artificial Intelligence and Computer Vision
(C) Both A and B

3. What is one application of Sign Language Processing mentioned in the chapter?

(A) Developing interactive educational tools
(B) Creating antivirus software
(C) Enhancing GPS technology

4. What system is used for practical writing for deaf sign languages?

(A) Stokoe Notation
(B) SignWriting
(C) HamNoSys

5. Which technique is NOT mentioned as used in sign language detection tasks?

(A) Skin Color Detection (SCD)
(B) Motion Detection
(C) Echo Location

6. What does the Sign Language Detection process initially identify in an image or video?

(A) If the content contains spoken language
(B) If the content contains sign language
(C) If the content contains textual information

7. What is the purpose of the Sign Language Classification stage mentioned in the chapter?

(A) To determine the emotional state of the signer
(B) To classify the identified sign language into specific types like ASL or BSL
(C) To translate sign language into spoken language directly

8. Which of the following is a focus of the cognitive mechanisms discussed in sign language processing?

(A) Effects of age of acquisition and iconicity
(B) Improving short-term memory
(C) Enhancing decision-making skills

9. What does the chapter indicate about the relationship between NLP and sign language processing?

(A) They are completely separate with no overlap
(B) They share goals of understanding and generating language
(C) Sign language processing is a subset of NLP focusing only on speech

10. What challenge is associated with sign language detection as discussed in the chapter?

(A) The simplicity of sign language gestures
(B) The intricate nature of sign language including factors like hand shapes and body postures
(C) The lack of visual components in sign language

References

1. Yin, K., Moryossef, A., Hochgesang, J., Goldberg, Y., Alikhani, M.: Including Signed Languages in Natural Language Processing, http://arxiv.org/abs/2105.05222, (2021).
2. Bragg, D., Koller, O., Bellard, M., Berke, L., Boudreault, P., Braffort, A., Caselli, N., Huenerfauth, M., Kacorri, H., Verhoef, T., Vogler, C., Ringel Morris, M.: Sign Language Recognition, Generation, and Translation: An Interdisciplinary Perspective. In: The 21st International ACM SIGACCESS Conference on Computers and Accessibility. pp. 16–31. ACM, Pittsburgh PA USA (2019). https://doi.org/10.1145/3308561.3353774.
3. Aran, O., Akarun, L.: Sign Language Processing and Interactive Tools for Sign Language Education. In: 2007 IEEE 15th Signal Processing and Communications Applications. pp. 1–4. IEEE, Eskisehir, Turkey (2007). https://doi.org/10.1109/SIU.2007.4298840.
4. Kamal, S.M., Chen, Y., Li, S., Shi, X., Zheng, J.: Technical Approaches to Chinese Sign Language Processing: A Review. IEEE Access. 7, 96926–96935 (2019). https://doi.org/10.1109/ACCESS.2019.2929174.

5. Carreiras, M.: Sign Language Processing. Language and Linguistics Compass. 4, 430–444 (2010). https://doi.org/10.1111/j.1749-818X.2010.00192.x.
6. Da Rocha Costa, A.C., Dimuro, G.P.: SignWriting-Based Sign Language Processing. In: Wachsmuth, I. and Sowa, T. (eds.) Gesture and Sign Language in Human-Computer Interaction. pp. 202–205. Springer Berlin Heidelberg, Berlin, Heidelberg (2002). https://doi.org/10.1007/3-540-47873-6_22.
7. Othman, A., Jemni, M.: Designing high accuracy statistical machine translation for sign language using parallel corpus: case study English and American Sign Language. Journal of Information Technology Research (JITR). 12, 134–158 (2019).
8. Iyer, V.H., Prakash, U.M., Vijay, A., Sathishkumar, P.: Sign Language Detection using Action Recognition. In: 2022 2nd International Conference on Advance Computing and Innovative Technologies in Engineering (ICACITE). pp. 1682–1685. IEEE, Greater Noida, India (2022). https://doi.org/10.1109/ICACITE53722.2022.9823484.
9. Patil, K., Pendharkar, G., Gaikwad, G.N.: American Sign Language Detection. 4, (2014).
10. Deep, A., Litoriya, A., Ingole, A., Asare, V., Bhole, S.M., Pathak, S.: Realtime Sign Language Detection and Recognition. In: 2022 2nd Asian Conference on Innovation in Technology (ASIANCON). pp. 1–4. IEEE, Ravet, India (2022). https://doi.org/10.1109/ASIANCON55314.2022.9908995.
11. Mondhe, D., Patil, R., Jadhav, V., Agarwal, P., Cs, L.: Sign Detect: An app to detect sign language. In: 2022 IEEE International Conference on Metrology for Extended Reality, Artificial Intelligence and Neural Engineering (MetroXRAINE). pp. 11–15. IEEE, Rome, Italy (2022). https://doi.org/10.1109/MetroXRAINE54828.2022.9967529.
12. Kawulok, M.: Dynamic Skin Detection in Color Images for Sign Language Recognition. In: Elmoataz, A., Lezoray, O., Nouboud, F., and Mammass, D. (eds.) Image and Signal Processing. pp. 112–119. Springer Berlin Heidelberg, Berlin, Heidelberg (2008). https://doi.org/10.1007/978-3-540-69905-7_13.
13. Konwar, A.S., Borah, B.S., Tuithung, C.T.: An American Sign Language detection system using HSV color model and edge detection. In: 2014 International Conference on Communication and Signal Processing. pp. 743–747. IEEE, Melmaruvathur, India (2014). https://doi.org/10.1109/ICCSP.2014.6949942.
14. Khan, S., Ali, M.E., Das, S.S., Rahman, M.M.: Real Time Hand Gesture Recognition by Skin Color Detection for American Sign Language. In: 2019 4th International Conference on Electrical Information and Communication Technology (EICT). pp. 1–6. IEEE, Khulna, Bangladesh (2019). https://doi.org/10.1109/EICT48899.2019.9068809.
15. Paulraj, M.P., Yaacob, S., Bin Zanar Azalan, M.S., Palaniappan, R.: A phoneme based sign language recognition system using skin color segmentation. In: 2010 6th International Colloquium on Signal Processing & its Applications. pp. 1–5. IEEE, Mallaca City (2010). https://doi.org/10.1109/CSPA.2010.5545253.
16. Dhanjal, A.S., Singh, W.: Comparative Analysis of Sign Language Notation Systems for Indian Sign Language. In: 2019 Second International Conference on Advanced Computational and Communication Paradigms (ICACCP). pp. 1–6. IEEE, Gangtok, India (2019). https://doi.org/10.1109/ICACCP.2019.8883009.
17. Miller, C.: Sign Language: Transcription, Notation, and Writing. In: Encyclopedia of Language & Linguistics. pp. 353–354. Elsevier (2006). https://doi.org/10.1016/B0-08-044854-2/00242-X.
18. Koizumi, A., Sagawa, H., Takeuchi, M.: An Annotated Japanese Sign Language Corpus. In: González Rodríguez, M. and Suarez Araujo, C.P. (eds.) Proceedings of the Third International Conference on Language Resources and Evaluation (LREC'02). European Language Resources Association (ELRA), Las Palmas, Canary Islands - Spain (2002).
19. Dubot, R., Collet, C.: A hybrid formalism to parse Sign Languages, http://arxiv.org/abs/1403.4467, (2014).
20. Chaaban, H., Gouiffès, M., Braffort, A.: Automatic Annotation and Segmentation of Sign Language Videos: Base-level Features and Lexical Signs Classification. In: 16th International Joint Conference on Computer Vision, Imaging and Computer Graphics Theory

and Applications (VISIGRAPP 2021). pp. 484–491. Online streaming, France (2021). 10.5220/0010247104840491.
21. Schembri, A. and Crasborn, O., 2010, May. Issues in creating annotation standards for sign language description. In sign-lang@ LREC 2010 (pp. 212-216). European Language Resources Association (ELRA).
22. Sallandre, M.-A., Garcia, B.: Epistemological issues in the semiological model for the annotation of sign languages. In: Meurant, L., Sinte, A., Van Herreweghe, M., and Vermeerbergen, M. (eds.) Sign Language Research, Uses and Practices. pp. 159–178. DE GRUYTER (2013). https://doi.org/10.1515/9781614511472.159.
23. Aitpayev, K., Islam, S., Imashev, A.: Semi-automatic annotation tool for sign languages. In: 2016 IEEE 10th International Conference on Application of Information and Communication Technologies (AICT). pp. 1–4. IEEE, Baku, Azerbaijan (2016). https://doi.org/10.1109/ICAICT.2016.7991803.
24. Dreuw, P., Ney, H.: Towards Automatic Sign Language Annotation for the ELAN Tool. In: Proceedings of the LREC2008 3rd Workshop on the Representation and Processing of Sign Languages: Construction and Exploitation of Sign Language Corpora. pp. 50–53. European Language Resources Association (ELRA), Marrakech, Morocco (2008).
25. Othman, A., Jemni, M.: An XML-gloss annotation system for sign language processing. In: 2017 6th International Conference on Information and Communication Technology and Accessibility (ICTA). pp. 1–7. IEEE, Muscat, Oman (2017). https://doi.org/10.1109/ICTA.2017.8336054.
26. Chételat-Pelé, E., Braffort, A.: Sign Language Corpus Annotation: toward a new Methodology. In: Calzolari, N., Choukri, K., Maegaard, B., Mariani, J., Odijk, J., Piperidis, S., and Tapias, D. (eds.) Proceedings of the Sixth International Conference on Language Resources and Evaluation (LREC'08). European Language Resources Association (ELRA), Marrakech, Morocco (2008).
27. Cormier, K.A., Crasborn, O., Bank, R.: Digging into Signs: Emerging Annotation Standards for Sign Language Corpora, http://www.lrec-conf.org/proceedings/lrec2016/index.html, last accessed 2024/04/11.
28. Braffort, A., Choisier, A., Collet, C., Dalle, P., Gianni, F., Lenseigne, F., Segouat, J.: Toward an Annotation Software for Video of Sign Language, Including Image Processing Tools and Signing Space Modelling. In: Lino, M.T., Xavier, M.F., Ferreira, F., Costa, R., and Silva, R. (eds.) Proceedings of the Fourth International Conference on Language Resources and Evaluation (LREC'04). European Language Resources Association (ELRA), Lisbon, Portugal (2004).
29. Stokoe, W.C.: Sign Language Structure: An Outline of the Visual Communication Systems of the American Deaf. Journal of Deaf Studies and Deaf Education. 10, 3–37 (2005). https://doi.org/10.1093/deafed/eni001.
30. Brentari, D.: A prosodic model of sign language phonology. MIT Press, Cambridge, Mass (1998).
31. Skobov, V., Lepage, Y.: Video-to-HamNoSys Automated Annotation System. In: Efthimiou, E., Fotinea, S.-E., Hanke, T., Hochgesang, J.A., Kristoffersen, J., and Mesch, J. (eds.) Proceedings of the LREC2020 9th Workshop on the Representation and Processing of Sign Languages: Sign Language Resources in the Service of the Language Community, Technological Challenges and Application Perspectives. pp. 209–216. European Language Resources Association (ELRA), Marseille, France (2020).
32. Takkinen, R.: Some observations on the use of HamNoSys (Hamburg Notation System for Sign Languages) in the context of the phonetic transcription of children's signing. SL&L. 8, 99–118 (2005). https://doi.org/10.1075/sll.8.1.05tak.
33. Majchrowska, S., Plantykow, M., Olech, M.: Handling sign language transcription system with the computer-friendly numerical multilabels. (2022). 10.48550/ARXIV.2204.06924.
34. Kanis, J., Krňoul, Z.: Interactive HamNoSys Notation Editor for Signed Speech Annotation. In: Proceedings of the LREC2008 3rd Workshop on the Representation and Processing of Sign Languages: Construction and Exploitation of Sign Language Corpora. pp. 88–93. European Language Resources Association (ELRA), Marrakech, Morocco (2008).

35. Koller, O., Bowden, R., Ney, H.: Automatic Alignment of HamNoSys Subunits for Continuous Sign Language Recognition. Presented at the May 1 (2016).
36. Kaur, K., Kumar, P.: HamNoSys to SiGML Conversion System for Sign Language Automation. Procedia Computer Science. 89, 794–803 (2016). https://doi.org/10.1016/j.procs.2016.06.063.
37. Kato, M.: A Study of Notation and Sign Writing Systems for the Deaf. Presented at the (2008).
38. Matsumoto, T., Kato, M., Ikeda, T.: JSPad: a sign language writing tool using SignWriting. In: Proceedings of the 3rd International Universal Communication Symposium. pp. 363–367. ACM, Tokyo Japan (2009). https://doi.org/10.1145/1667780.1667855.
39. Stiehl, D., Addams, L., Oliveira, L.S., Guimaraes, C., Britto, A.S.: Towards a SignWriting recognition system. In: 2015 13th International Conference on Document Analysis and Recognition (ICDAR). pp. 26–30. IEEE, Tunis, Tunisia (2015). https://doi.org/10.1109/ICDAR.2015.7333719.
40. Bouzid, Y., Jemni, M.: tuniSigner: A Virtual Interpreter to Learn Sign Writing. In: 2014 IEEE 14th International Conference on Advanced Learning Technologies. pp. 601–605. IEEE, Athens, Greece (2014). https://doi.org/10.1109/ICALT.2014.176.
41. Ormel, E., Crasborn, O., Kooij, E.V.D., Dijken, L. van, Nauta, Y.E., Forster, J., Stein, D.: Glossing a multi-purpose sign language corpus. Presented at the International Conference on Language Resources and Evaluation (2010).
42. Mesch, J., Wallin, L.: Gloss annotations in the Swedish Sign Language Corpus. IJCL. 20, 102–120 (2015). https://doi.org/10.1075/ijcl.20.1.05mes.
43. Antinoro Pizzuto, E., Pietrandrea, P.: The notation of signed texts: Open questions and indications for further research. SL&L. 4, 29–45 (2001). https://doi.org/10.1075/sll.4.12.05piz.
44. Aouiti, N., Jemni, M., Semreen, S.: Arab gloss annotation system for Arabic Sign Language. In: 2015 5th International Conference on Information & Communication Technology and Accessibility (ICTA). pp. 1–6. IEEE, Marrakech (2015). https://doi.org/10.1109/ICTA.2015.7426932.
45. Jemni, M., Semreen, S., Othman, A., Tmar, Z., Aouiti, N.: Toward the creation of an Arab Gloss for arabic Sign Language annotation. In: Fourth International Conference on Information and Communication Technology and Accessibility (ICTA). pp. 1–5. IEEE, Hammamet, Tunisia (2013). https://doi.org/10.1109/ICTA.2013.6815292.
46. Hanke, T., König, L., Konrad, R., Kopf, M., Schulder, M., Wolfe, R.: Easier Notation – a Proposal for a Gloss-Based Scripting Language for Sign Language Generation Based on Lexical Data. In: 2023 IEEE International Conference on Acoustics, Speech, and Signal Processing Workshops (ICASSPW). pp. 1–5. IEEE, Rhodes Island, Greece (2023). https://doi.org/10.1109/ICASSPW59220.2023.10192997.
47. Hall, K.C., Aonuki, Y., Vesik, K., Poy, A., Tolmie, N.: Sign Language Phonetic Annotator-Analyzer: Open-Source Software for Form-Based Analysis of Sign Languages. In: Proceedings of the LREC2022 10th Workshop on the Representation and Processing of Sign Languages: Multilingual Sign Language Resources. pp. 59–66. European Language Resources Association (ELRA), Marseille, France (2022).
48. Othman, A., El Ghoul, O., Aziz, M., Chemnad, K., Sedrati, S., Dhouib, A.: JUMLA-QSL-22: Creation and Annotation of a Qatari Sign Language Corpus for Sign Language Processing. In: Proceedings of the 16th International Conference on PErvasive Technologies Related to Assistive Environments. pp. 686–692 (2023).
49. El Ghoul, O.E.G., Othman, A.O., Aziz, M.A., Sedrati, S.S.: JUMLA-QSL-22: A dataset of Qatari sign language sentences, https://ieee-dataport.org/open-access/jumla-qsl-22-dataset-qatari-sign-language-sentences. 10.21227/CKZP-3754.
50. Mukushev, M., Kydyrbekova, A., Kimmelman, V., Sandygulova, A.: Towards Large Vocabulary Kazakh-Russian Sign Language Dataset: KRSL-OnlineSchool. In: Efthimiou, E., Fotinea, S.-E., Hanke, T., Hochgesang, J.A., Kristoffersen, J., Mesch, J., and Schulder, M. (eds.) Proceedings of the LREC2022 10th Workshop on the Representation and Processing of Sign Languages: Multilingual Sign Language Resources. pp. 154–158. European Language Resources Association, Marseille, France (2022).

Chapter 6
Advanced Sign Language Tasks

6.1 Introduction

This chapter on Sign Language Processing (SLP), part 2, builds upon the foundational discussions introduced in Chap. 5, focusing on further essential tasks within the SLP framework as presented in Fig. 6.1.

This chapter examines several key processes crucial to the advancement of this field. We begin by exploring Sign Language Segmentation, which involves dividing continuous sign language input into distinct signs or phrases, setting the stage for more detailed analysis. The discussion extends to Sign Language Clustering, which categorizes similar signs together, simplifying complexity for subsequent recognition tasks. The section on Sign Language Recognition addresses the interpretation of segmented signs into forms understandable by both machines and humans. This section will introduce the methods and technologies used to enhance accuracy and efficiency in recognition systems. Following this, we will discuss Sign Language Translation, focusing on converting sign language into spoken or written text. This process is vital for facilitating communication between Deaf and hearing individuals. Finally, we address Sign Language Generation, where spoken or written language is converted back into sign language, often using avatars or animated figures.

6.2 Sign Language Spotting

Sign language spotting or segmentation breaks down a continuous stream of sign language into its constituent signs or phrases (see Fig. 6.1). This is a critical step in sign language processing, allowing for the subsequent detailed analysis and understanding of the content. The process involves several stages and employs various

A. Othman, *Sign Language Processing*,
https://doi.org/10.1007/978-3-031-68763-1_6

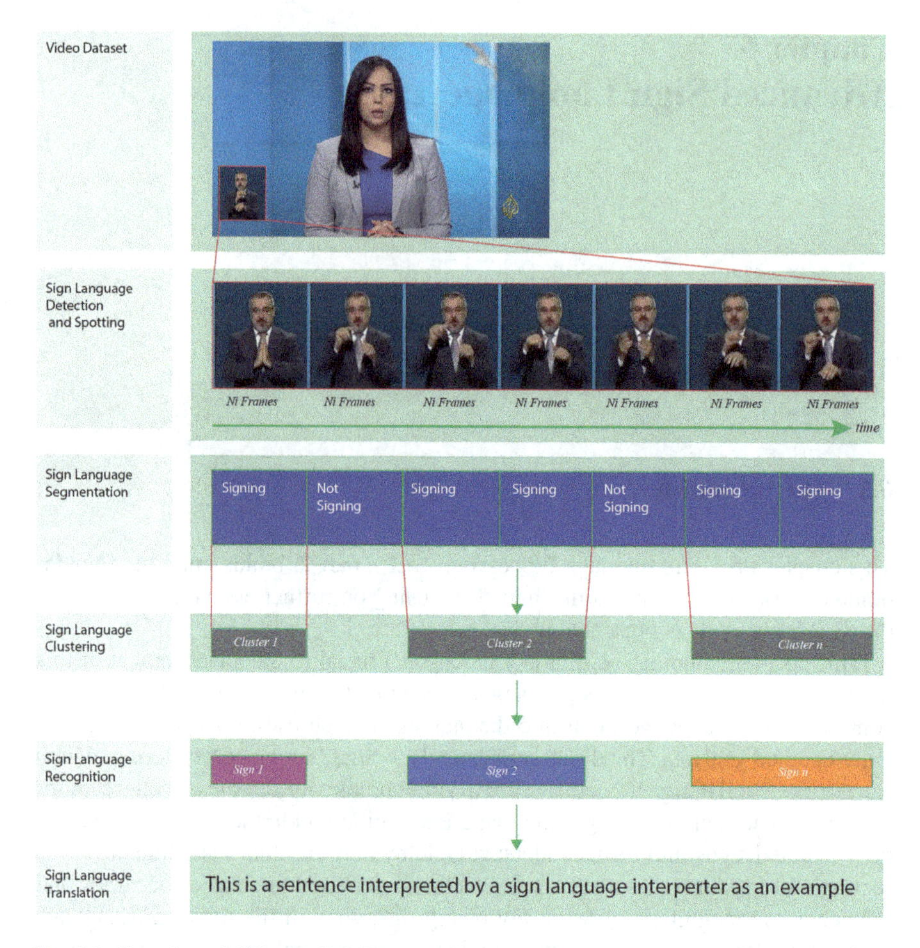

Fig. 6.1 Overview of different SLP Tasks applied on a video from YouTube (News Video from AlJazeera YouTube Channel: https://youtu.be/_5UFETOCurQ)

technologies and methods to segment the sign language input accurately and efficiently.

The first step in sign language spotting is identifying the beginning and end of a sign or phrase. This often relies on motion detection techniques, where periods of minimal motion may indicate pauses between signs. Advanced computer vision algorithms track movements, focusing on the hands and face, to determine when a sign starts and stops.

Machine learning models, particularly those involving time-series analysis, are extensively used to predict transitions between signs. Models such as hidden Markov Models (HMMs) and Recurrent Neural Networks (RNNs), including Long-Short-Term Memory networks (LSTMs), are trained on labeled datasets of sign language videos to learn the temporal dynamics characteristic of sign language.

Non-manual elements such as facial expressions and body posture are integral to understanding the structure of sign language. The segmentation process often incorporates these features to differentiate between signs with similar hand movements but different meanings based on the accompanying non-manual signals.

Computer vision plays a significant role in the segmentation process. Techniques such as optical flow, which tracks the movement of objects (e.g., hands) between frames, and skin color detection, which helps isolate the hands and face from the rest of the image, are common. These methods enhance the model's ability to segment the video accurately by focusing analysis on the most relevant parts of the frame.

Recently, deep learning approaches have been applied to improve the accuracy of sign language segmentation. Convolutional Neural Networks (CNNs) and RNNs are combined to extract spatial features from individual frames and temporal features across sequences. This combination is particularly effective in capturing the complex patterns of movement that characterize sign language.

After the initial segmentation, post-processing steps are often necessary to refine the segment boundaries. These may include smoothing techniques to ensure the segments are coherently defined and adjusting the start and end points based on refined criteria such as minimal hand movement.

Segmentation of sign language presents unique challenges. Variability in signing speed, style, and space used by different signers can affect the performance of segmentation algorithms. Additionally, the quality of input data, such as video resolution and lighting conditions, impacts the segmentation process.

A concrete example of good practice in sign language spotting or segmentation is presented in the work of Enriquez et al. in 2022 [1] as a challenge. The ECCV 2022 Sign Spotting Challenge[1] significantly advances sign language segmentation, particularly in continuous sign language recognition. This challenge introduced a new dataset specifically designed for fine-grain sign spotting within the health domain of Spanish Sign Language, comprising approximately 10 h of video data annotated by experts. This dataset is unique due to its frame-level precise annotation of signs, facilitating the development and testing of sign language segmentation algorithms under controlled conditions.

A key aspect of this challenge was its focus on developing technologies that can accurately identify and segment signs from a continuous flow, considering the co-articulation effects and the variability in the realization of signs. The challenge highlighted the effectiveness of advanced machine learning models, including deep learning frameworks that utilize spatial-temporal data representation. Participants employed innovative approaches such as 3DCNNs and ST-GCNs to tackle the complexities of segmenting signs intricately integrated into fluent signing.

This exploration into fine-grained sign spotting and segmentation underscores the potential of these technologies to enhance the accessibility of sign language content by enabling precise search functionalities and aiding educational tools. The challenge's outcomes demonstrate a significant step forward in making sign language content more navigable and understandable, thus contributing positively to linguistics and accessibility technology.

---

[1] About the challenge: https://chalearnlap.cvc.uab.cat/challenge/49/description/

Definition Sign language spotting or segmentation is a task in computational linguistics that identifies and locates specific signs within continuous streams of sign language. It focuses on detecting particular signs accurately and determining their temporal boundaries, utilizing advanced machine learning and computer vision techniques.

6.3 Sign Language Clustering

Sign language clustering is a technique used in computational linguistics to group similar signs together, facilitating more efficient recognition and analysis of sign language data. This approach is instrumental in managing the inherent diversity in sign language, where variations in expression, speed, and style can significantly impact recognition.

Sign language clustering involves categorizing signs that share standard features into clusters. By doing so, the recognition system can treat each cluster as a singular entity during the initial processing stages, simplifying the recognition task by reducing the complexity and variability it must handle simultaneously.

Definition Sign language clustering is the process of grouping similar signs together in sign language data to simplify recognition tasks, identify anomalies, and align signs with semantic meanings for more accurate interpretation and translation.

Several techniques can be used for sign language clustering, each bringing a unique approach to handling the complexity and variability inherent in sign language data. Clustering algorithms are crucial for grouping similar signs, facilitating more efficient recognition, and enhancing the interpretability of sign language within computational models. Here are some of the primary techniques employed:

- **K-means Clustering**: This algorithm is popular for partitioning a dataset into a fixed number (k) of clusters. It defines centroids, one for each cluster, and then assigns each data point (sign) to the nearest centroid. The process iterates, recalculating centroids and reassigning points until minimal change occurs in the cluster assignments. This method is beneficial when the clusters are expected to be roughly spherical and evenly sized.
- **Hierarchical Clustering**: Unlike K-means, hierarchical clustering does not require a pre-specified number of clusters. It builds a hierarchy of clusters either through an agglomerative (bottom-up) approach, where each observation starts in its cluster and pairs of clusters are merged as one moves up the hierarchy, or a divisive (top-down) approach, where all observations start in one cluster. Splits are performed recursively as one moves down the hierarchy. The result is a tree-based representation of the observations, called a dendrogram, which helps visualize the data's clustering structure.
- **DBSCAN (Density-Based Spatial Clustering of Applications with Noise)**: This algorithm groups together closely packed points while marking points that lie alone in low-density regions as outliers. DBSCAN is particularly suited for

sign language data due to its ability to handle clusters of arbitrary shape and size, which is often the case with the diverse manifestations of signs.

- **Spectral Clustering**: Utilizing the spectrum (eigenvalues) of the data's similarity matrix, spectral clustering can perform dimensionality reduction before clustering in fewer dimensions. This method is effective when the clusters' structure is highly non-convex or more complex than just spherical, as in k-means.
- **Feature Extraction with Deep Learning**: Techniques such as autoencoders or convolutional neural networks can extract meaningful features from sign language video data. These features, which may capture subtle aspects of hand shape, motion, and expression not easily categorized by more straightforward clustering methods, can then be clustered using any of the above methods to form meaningful groups.
- **Self-Organizing Maps (SOMs)**: SOMs are an artificial neural network trained using unsupervised learning to produce a low-dimensional (typically two-dimensional), discretized representation of the input space of the training samples. This method helps visualize high-dimensional data and can help identify patterns and clusters within sign language datasets.
- **Agglomerative Information Bottleneck (AIB)**: This technique focuses on clustering data points to maximize the mutual information between input variables and clusters. It's handy for situations where preserving information content during clustering is critical, such as in sign language interpretation, where the loss of subtle sign features could lead to significant changes in meaning.

Sign language clustering finds its usefulness in several applications across different fields. Here are some extended examples:

- **Enhanced Recognition Systems**: Clustering in sign language recognition systems significantly reduces computational complexity. By grouping similar signs into clusters, recognition algorithms can process these groups rather than individually, considerably speeding up the recognition process and reducing resource consumption.
- **Anomaly Detection**: In data analysis, clustering helps identify signs that deviate from the norm. These anomalies may indicate rare variations of signs or potential errors in sign interpretation. Detecting such anomalies is crucial for systems that rely on high accuracy, such as educational software or communicative technologies used by the deaf community.
- **Semantic Analysis**: Clustering signs based on their semantic content allows for more nuanced interpretation and translation of sign language. By understanding which signs convey similar meanings or emotions, systems can provide more contextually appropriate translations, enhancing the quality of communication between sign language users and the broader public.
- **Educational Tools**: Sign language clustering can help create more effective learning modules in educational settings. By grouping signs with standard features or meanings, educational tools can offer targeted lessons that progressively teach sign language, building from simple to more complex groups of signs.

- **Content Indexing and Search**: In digital archives of sign language content, clustering facilitates efficient search and indexing by categorizing signs into easily navigable groups. Users searching for specific content can quickly locate relevant signs and videos, making digital libraries more user-friendly.
- **Linguistic Research**: Researchers studying the structure and usage of sign languages benefit from clustering by being able to analyze how certain signs are related or differ from one another. This can lead to new insights into the evolution of sign language and its regional variations.

In sign language segmentation, several metrics are employed to evaluate the accuracy and efficiency of segmentation algorithms. These metrics help determine how well a model can isolate and identify individual signs from continuous sign language streams. Here are some of the key metrics commonly used (Table 6.1):

Table 6.1 Example of metrics used in sign language segmentation

Metric name	Description
Intersection over Union (IoU)	Known as the Jaccard index, this metric is widely used in computer vision and is particularly crucial in tasks involving object detection and segmentation. IoU measures the overlap between the predicted and ground truth segmentation, expressed as the ratio of their intersection to their union. Sign language segmentation quantifies how accurately the signs are segmented compared to manually segmented ground truth.
F1 Score	This is the harmonic mean of precision and recall. Precision measures the accuracy of the optimistic predictions (i.e., the proportion of correctly segmented signs out of all segments identified by the model as signs). In contrast, recall measures the ability to find all the relevant instances (i.e., the proportion of actual signs correctly identified by the model). The F1 score is instrumental in sign language segmentation because it balances both precision and recall, providing a single measure to evaluate the model's overall performance.
Accuracy	This metric calculates the proportion of correctly segmented frames over the total number of frames. Accuracy is straightforward and provides a quick snapshot of the model's effectiveness. However, it may not always be the best standalone metric, especially if the data is imbalanced (i.e., the number of non-sign frames significantly outnumbers the sign frames).
Mean Squared Error (MSE)	In scenarios where temporal boundaries are predicted as continuous values, MSE can be used to measure the average squared difference between the estimated values and the actual values. MSE clearly indicates the precision of boundary predictions in temporal segmentation tasks.
Recall Rate at False Accept Rate (FAR)	This metric is used mainly in detection tasks where the trade-off between detecting true positives and avoiding false positives is critical. It measures how many actual positive cases are correctly identified while keeping the false positives below a certain threshold.
Frame-wise Classification Accuracy	This metric assesses the accuracy of models that perform frame-by-frame segmentation on a frame-wise basis. It checks whether each frame is correctly classified as part of a sign, providing detailed insight into the model's performance at a granular level.

6.4 Sign Language Recognition

Sign language recognition (SLR) is a branch of computational linguistics and computer vision focusing on interpreting and translating sign language into text or speech. This complex field requires the integration of various technologies to accurately process and understand the nuances of sign language, which is inherently visual and spatial. Below is a comprehensive overview of SLR, covering the interpretation of segmented signs, the technologies involved, the challenges faced, and the transformation of signs into formats that are understandable by both machines and humans.

In SLR, the first step typically involves segmenting continuous sign language footage into individual signs or phrases. This segmentation is crucial as it isolates distinct elements of the sign language stream, making it easier for the subsequent recognition algorithms to process each segment independently. Once segmented, each sign or phrase undergoes a detailed interpretation process where the movement, hand shape, orientation, and facial expressions are analyzed to determine the meaning. This interpretation relies heavily on the contextual understanding of how different signs relate to each other within a sentence or phrase.

SLR employs various techniques to interpret and translate sign language effectively. These techniques often involve a combination of computer vision, machine learning, and sensor technologies. Figure 6.2 is an overview of the primary methods used in SLR.

Definition Sign language recognition (SLR) is the technological process of identifying and interpreting sign language gestures using computational methods, translating them into text or spoken language to facilitate communication between deaf and hearing individuals.

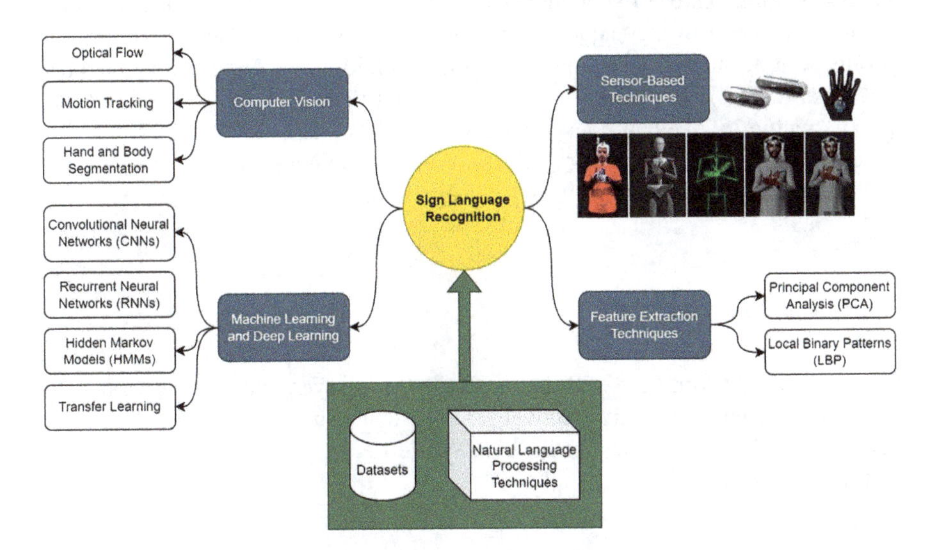

Fig. 6.2 Overview of different sign language recognition techniques

Skeleton Aware Multi-modal Sign Language Recognition Technique

In the work of Jiang et al. [2], The "Skeleton Aware Multi-modal Sign Language Recognition Technique" represents a sophisticated approach in the field of SLR, leveraging the strengths of multi-modal data inputs and advanced computational frameworks to enhance the accuracy and robustness of sign language interpretation. This technique integrates multiple data inputs, notably skeleton data, which refers to the 3D positions of body joints. These inputs can be derived from depth cameras or sensor-equipped suits that accurately capture the dynamic movements of a signer's body, hands, and face. Focusing on skeleton data effectively captures the nuances of sign language gestures, which are critical for accurate recognition.

In addition to skeleton data, the multi-modal aspect typically incorporates:

- Visual data (RGB): Standard video footage that provides detailed visual information about the signer's appearance and background context.
- Depth data: Offers 3D information about the spatial relationships and movements of the signer.
- Infrared data: Useful in low-light conditions and for enhancing the depth data accuracy.
- These diverse data streams are integrated to provide a comprehensive dataset that is processed by the recognition system, making the technique robust against variations in lighting, background, and signer positioning.

The technique primarily utilizes advanced deep learning models to enhance sign language recognition. Convolutional Neural Networks (CNNs) are pivotal for processing static images and extracting critical features from RGB data that highlight the visual complexities of sign language. RNNs and LSTMs manage the temporal dynamics inherent in the sequence of signs, ensuring the flow and continuity of gestures are accurately interpreted over time. Additionally, Graph Convolutional Networks (GCNs) are utilized to process skeletal data effectively, leveraging the graph structure of skeletal connections where joints and bones act as nodes and edges, thereby facilitating a comprehensive understanding of spatial relationships and movements crucial for precise sign recognition.

Evaluation Technique

Evaluating the performance of SLR systems involves several vital metrics that help assess how accurately and effectively the system can interpret sign language. Table 6.2 Evaluation Metrics for Sign Language Recognition presents the primary metrics used for this purpose.

Table 6.2 Evaluation metrics for sign language recognition

Metric	Description	Example of use	Formula
Accuracy	Measures the overall correctness of the model.	Evaluating the percentage of signs correctly recognized in a dataset.	$P = \frac{TP+TN}{TP+TN+FP+FN}$
Precision	Ratio of correctly predicted positive observations to the total predicted positives.	Used when the cost of false positives is high.	$P = \frac{TP}{TP+FP}$
Recall (sensitivity)	Measures the ability to identify all relevant instances.	Crucial in medical or safety applications where missing a sign is critical.	$P = \frac{TP}{TP+FN}$
F1 Score	Harmonic mean of Precision and Recall.	Balancing precision and recall, especially when classes are imbalanced.	$P = 2 \times \frac{Precision \times Recall}{Precision + Recall}$
Intersection over Union (IoU)	Measures the overlap between predicted segmentation and ground truth.	Used in sign language video segmentation to assess the accuracy of each segmented sign.	$P = \frac{Area\ of\ Overlap}{Area\ of\ Union}$
Mean Squared Error (MSE)	Measures the average of the squares of the errors.	Used in predicting the temporal boundaries of signs within videos.	$P = \frac{1}{n}\sum_{i=1}^{n}\left(Y_i - \hat{Y}_i\right)^2$

Where: P—Evaluation Score, TP—True Positives, TN—True Negatives, FP—False Positives, FN—False Negatives

6.5 Sign Language Translation

Sign Language Translation (SLT) involves converting the visual-gestural modality of sign language into spoken or written language. This process is pivotal in bridging communication gaps between Deaf and hearing individuals, promoting inclusivity, and ensuring that Deaf individuals can participate fully in societal, educational, and professional settings.

The translation process starts with capturing and segmenting sign language through video or sensor-based inputs. Advanced camera systems or specialized wearable technology, such as data gloves and motion sensors, capture sign language's dynamic movements and nuances. This raw data is segmented into distinct signs or phrases, a critical step that involves delineating where one sign ends and another begins.

Once the signs are segmented, the next phase is sign language recognition, where each segmented sign is identified and classified. This step typically employs machine learning algorithms and computer vision techniques. CNNs are particularly effective for recognizing the spatial features of signs. At the same time, RNNs, including LSTMs, are used to handle the temporal sequences of sign language, as presented in the previous section.

Definition Sign Language Translation (SLT) is the process of converting sign language into spoken or written language, or vice versa, facilitating communication between Deaf and hearing individuals. This involves not only the direct translation of signs but also the adaptation of grammatical and contextual nuances to preserve the integrity and meaning of the original message.

Following recognition, the translation phase converts the recognized signs into equivalent spoken or written text (Fig. 6.3). This involves not just a direct translation of individual signs but also an interpretation of sign language's grammatical and syntactical structure, which differs significantly from spoken languages. Machine Translation (MT) systems, extensively developed for spoken and written languages, are adapted to handle the unique challenges of sign language structures. In the upcoming chapters, we will investigate MT for SL more. The translation of sign language to spoken or written language is crucial for several reasons:

- Accessibility: It ensures that Deaf individuals have access to information and communication in public life, including education, healthcare, and legal settings.

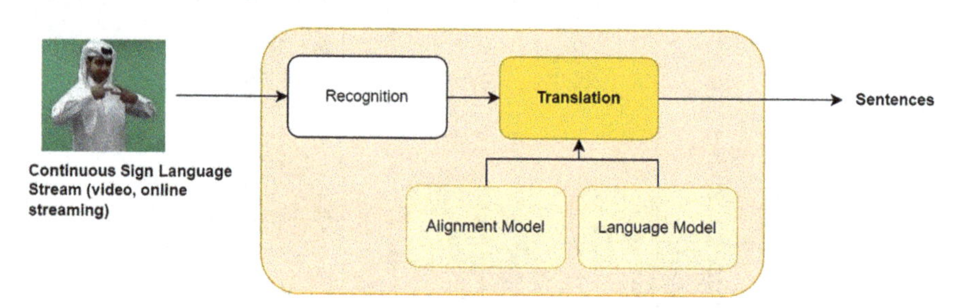

Fig. 6.3 Sign language translation pipeline

- Inclusivity: Effective communication support through translation facilitates the integration of Deaf individuals into the workforce and social groups, promoting inclusivity and diversity.
- Autonomy: By providing tools that can translate sign language, Deaf individuals are empowered to communicate independently without relying solely on human interpreters.
- Emergency Services: In emergency situations, quick and accurate translation can be life-saving, providing Deaf individuals the means to communicate effectively with emergency responders.

6.6 Sign Language Generation and Synthesis

The generation and synthesis of sign language from spoken or written text involve converting textual information into visual sign language representations, typically using digital avatars or animated figures. This process is crucial for providing accessibility solutions for the deaf and hard-of-hearing community, allowing them to receive information in their native sign language.

Virtual Conversation Agents (also called avatars) are a technology for displaying signed conversations without showing a video of a human signer. Instead, the systems use 3D animated models, which can be stored more efficiently than video. The avatar can move the fingers and hands, make facial gestures for facial expressions (happiness, surprise, etc.), body movements, and co-signs, in which two different words or ideas are signed at the same time. The avatar can be programmed to communicate in sign language (for example, in ASL or LSF). Advances in computer graphics capabilities mean that personal computers and smartphones can produce this animation with much greater clarity than in the past when transitions between the signs were rough and smooth, and the hands had to return to a central position between each sign.

Digital avatars that translate content or audio into sign language have a broad spectrum of applications, enhancing accessibility for the deaf and hard-of-hearing community across various sectors [3]. In educational settings, these avatars can be integrated into e-learning platforms to provide sign language translations of textual or spoken materials, making academic content more inclusive. Healthcare institutions can use avatars to translate medical information and patient instructions, ensuring that deaf patients receive critical health information in a format they can understand. Furthermore, public services, such as televised broadcasts or emergency announcements, can employ avatars to deliver important news and safety instructions in sign language, broadening communication reach to include those who rely on sign language for information. Additionally, customer service centers can use avatars to interact with deaf customers, providing a more engaging and accessible service experience. These applications foster inclusivity and promote independence and equal access to information for individuals within the deaf community. More example of real applications is shown in Fig. 6.4 using the avatar BuHamad developed by Mada Center Qatar [4].

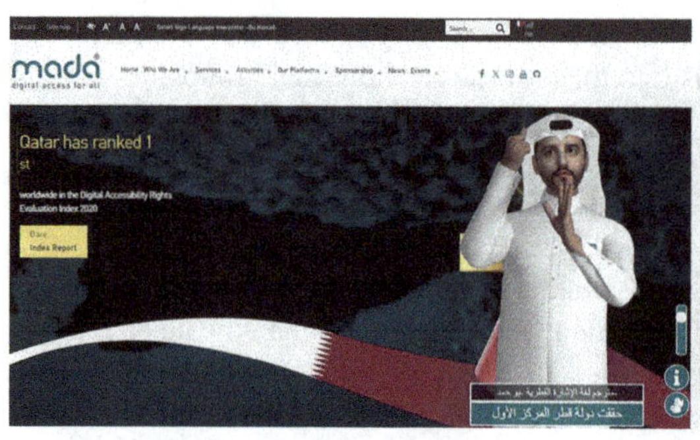

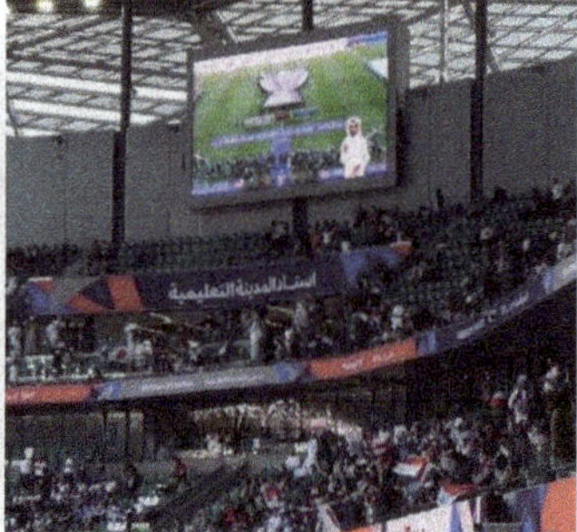

Fig. 6.4 Example of application using Avatar Technology to translate audio or text content into sign language (1) Mada Website (https://www.mada.org.qa) (2) Avatar BuHamad translating audio announcements inside stadiums in sign language during Asian Cup Qatar (https://www.instagram.com/buhamad.madacenter/) 2023

Definition Sign language Synthesis or Generation is the process of generating sign language expressions, typically using digital avatars or animated figures, from spoken or written language. This technology enables the conversion of text-based information into visual-gestural sign language, making content accessible to Deaf and hard-of-hearing audiences.

Implementing digital avatars for sign language translation presents several significant challenges that impact the technology's effectiveness and reliability. A primary concern is achieving the naturalness and fluidity of the avatar's movements, which is crucial for accurately portraying sign language's expressive nuances. Additionally, linguistic accuracy is paramount; errors in the avatar's signing could lead to misunderstandings or miscommunication, underscoring the need for precise modeling and animation.

Technical challenges also include real-time performance demands, where delays or lags in translation could disrupt the flow of communication, making live interactions and broadcasts less effective. Moreover, the need for avatars to be adaptable to various sign languages and customizable to different regional dialects adds complexity to the development process. Finally, conveying sign language's emotional and contextual subtleties through digital means requires sophisticated animation capabilities and deep linguistic insights, presenting ongoing developmental hurdles. These challenges highlight the intricate interplay of technology, linguistics, and user experience design necessary to develop and deploy effective sign language translation avatars.

6.7 Conclusion

In conclusion, this chapter has thoroughly explored the sophisticated realm of advanced sign language processing techniques, illustrating the depth and breadth of technological advancements in this field. We began by discussing the critical importance of sign language segmentation, a foundational step in the processing pipeline that involves dividing continuous streams of sign language into distinct, manageable units. This segmentation not only facilitates easier handling of the data but also sets the stage for more precise analysis in subsequent stages.

Following segmentation, we examined the role of sign language clustering. This technique groups similar signs together, simplifying the recognition tasks and enhancing the efficiency of the systems by reducing computational complexity. Clustering also aids in the preliminary categorization of signs, which is particularly beneficial for large datasets.

The recognition phase, which builds on the outputs of segmentation and clustering, involves identifying and interpreting the segmented signs. Here, advanced machine learning models and computer vision techniques come into play, demonstrating their capacity to effectively translate the visual information of sign language into data that computers can process and understand.

Further, we delved into translating sign language into spoken or written text—a vital process that bridges communication gaps between the Deaf and hearing communities. This translation is not only about converting signs into words but also involves preserving the grammatical and contextual integrity of the original language in the translated output.

Lastly, the generation of sign language from text, utilizing digital avatars and animated figures, was discussed. This process reverses the direction of sign language translation, demonstrating how textual or spoken information can be rendered into sign language, thus providing accessible content for the Deaf community.

Throughout the chapter, the intersection of technology with linguistic accuracy has been a recurring theme, emphasizing the need for continual improvements in both areas to enhance the effectiveness of sign language processing systems. The integration of these advanced techniques represents a significant step forward in making everyday communication more inclusive and accessible for the Deaf community, ultimately fostering greater understanding and interaction across different communication modalities.

Quiz Time

1. What is the first step in sign language spotting, as discussed in this chapter?

(A) Identifying non-manual elements
(B) Translation into spoken language
(C) Identification of the beginning and end of a sign or phrase

2. Which technology is commonly used in the segmentation of sign language?

(A) Optical flow
(B) Echo location
(C) Ultrasonic sensors

3. What role do machine learning models play in sign language segmentation?

(A) They predict transitions between signs.
(B) They convert signs into spoken language.
(C) They generate new sign language data.

4. Which models are mentioned as being used in time-series analysis for sign language?

(A) Linear Regression Models
(B) Hidden Markov Models and Recurrent Neural Networks
(C) Decision Tree Models

5. What is a key aspect of the ECCV 2022 Sign Spotting Challenge?

(A) It focuses on Spanish Sign Language.
(B) It uses only manual signs for spotting.
(C) It is limited to English Sign Language.

6. What is 'Sign Language Clustering' primarily used in computational linguistics?

(A) To group similar signs to simplify recognition tasks.
(B) To translate sign language into spoken language.
(C) To generate synthetic sign language data.

7. What method is not listed as a technique used for sign language clustering?

(A) K-means Clustering
(B) Hierarchical Clustering
(C) Binary Search

8. According to the chapter, what does sign language recognition involve?

(A) Translating text to sign language
(B) Identifying and interpreting segmented signs
(C) Clustering similar signs into groups

9. What does the 'Skeleton Aware Multi-modal Sign Language Recognition Technique' utilize for recognition?

(A) Only RGB data
(B) Only depth data
(C) Multiple types of data, including RGB, depth, and skeleton data

10. What challenge is associated with sign language generation using avatars, as discussed in the chapter?

(A) Making the avatars perform in real-time without lags
(B) Teaching avatars multiple sign languages
(C) Ensuring avatars can perform complex mathematical calculations

References

1. Vázquez Enríquez, M., Castro, J.L.A., Fernandez, L.D., Jacques Junior, J.C.S., Escalera, S.: ECCV 2022 Sign Spotting Challenge: Dataset, Design and Results. In: Karlinsky, L., Michaeli, T., and Nishino, K. (eds.) Computer Vision – ECCV 2022 Workshops. pp. 225–242. Springer Nature Switzerland, Cham (2023). https://doi.org/10.1007/978-3-031-25085-9_13.
2. Jiang, S., Sun, B., Wang, L., Bai, Y., Li, K., Fu, Y.: Skeleton Aware Multi-modal Sign Language Recognition. In: 2021 IEEE/CVF Conference on Computer Vision and Pattern Recognition Workshops (CVPRW). pp. 3408–3418 (2021). 10.1109/CVPRW53098.2021.00380.
3. Aziz, M., Othman, A.: Evolution and Trends in Sign Language Avatar Systems: Unveiling a 40-Year Journey via Systematic Review. Multimodal Technologies and Interaction. 7, 97 (2023).
4. Othman, A., El Ghoul, O.: BuHamad: The first Qatari virtual interpreter for Qatari Sign Language. Nafath. 6, (2022).

Chapter 7
Building Sign Language Datasets

7.1 Introduction

The construction and availability of datasets are foundational to progress in the broad spectrum of linguistic and computational research. Datasets provide crucial insight into the intricate dynamics of languages, enabling researchers to analyze, interpret, and advance our understanding of linguistic phenomena. This is especially pertinent in sign languages, where comprehensive datasets are indispensable. They serve as a rich repository of visual-spatial linguistic data, as investigated in Chap. 1, and drive the development of computational models and underpin significant technological advancements.

The previous chapters have highlighted various aspects of sign language processing, including identification, notation, annotation, segmentation, recognition, translation, and synthesis, underscoring the need for robust datasets. Effective sign language processing relies heavily on the quality and comprehensiveness of these datasets. Unlike spoken languages, which benefit from extensive textual corpora, sign languages present unique challenges due to their inherently visual and spatial nature. Accurately capturing the complex interplay of handshapes, movements, facial expressions, and other nuances is essential, necessitating datasets beyond mere text to include visual and often three-dimensional representations.

Building sign language datasets transcends the technical challenges of capturing and structuring data; it fundamentally involves deep cultural and community engagement. The Deaf and signing communities from which this data is drawn are not mere data points but vibrant collectives with rich cultural narratives and diverse experiences. Each dataset curated has the potential to reflect and respect these unique cultural dimensions, making ethical considerations and community involvement paramount.

Creating these datasets must be conducted with a high degree of sensitivity and inclusivity, ensuring that the methods employed extract information and contribute

A. Othman, *Sign Language Processing*,
https://doi.org/10.1007/978-3-031-68763-1_7

positively back to the community. This involves engaging with community members not just as participants but as collaborators who have a say in how their language and gestures are recorded, represented, and shared. Such participatory approaches help build trust and ensure that the datasets are comprehensive, culturally congruent, and respectful of the community's identity and privacy.

Furthermore, it is essential to consider how these datasets, once created, are used. Sign language representation in computational models must avoid perpetuating stereotypes or misrepresentations that could potentially harm the community. Instead, it should aim to elevate and amplify the linguistic diversity and cultural richness of the Deaf community. By integrating community feedback and adhering to strict ethical standards, creating sign language datasets can be a respectful and enriching process, benefiting the academic and Deaf communities in meaningful ways.

Definition A dataset is a structured collection of data, typically organized in a table format with rows and columns, where each row represents an individual record and columns represent the attributes or variables of the data. Datasets compile, store, and analyze information across various fields as the foundation for statistical analysis and predictive modeling.

This chapter will explore building sign language datasets' technical and ethical considerations. We will discuss the anatomy of these datasets, detailing the processes involved in data collection, storage, notation, and annotation. By examining best practices, challenges, and innovative solutions, this chapter sheds light on how effectively curated datasets can transform the landscape of sign language research and technology, enhancing communication and accessibility for the Deaf community.

7.2 What Is a Sign Language Dataset?

At its essence, a dataset is a meticulously organized collection of data, representing a structured and accessible format of raw information poised for detailed examination, analysis, and interpretation. This definition takes on a vivid dimension when applied to the domain of sign languages, where a dataset becomes an elaborate array of dynamic movements, facial expressions, and spatial interactions. In sign languages, a dataset captures the complex choreography of hands, facial expressions, and body movements that coalesce to create meaning through visual-spatial modalities.

Contrasting sharply with textual datasets used for spoken languages—which linearly arrange words and sentences—a sign language dataset encompasses sequences of visual gestures that communicate far beyond the mere verbal equivalents. These datasets are not limited to simple video recordings of sign language communication. They often extend to sophisticated data compilations that include three-dimensional motion capture, which records the precise movements of a signer's hands and body in space. Additionally, these datasets may feature depth-sensing information, providing crucial insights into the spatial aspects of sign language gestures and comprehensive annotations that describe each gesture in terms of its linguistic and semantic components.

Therefore, a typical sign language dataset might include extensive video libraries capturing a wide array of signers from diverse backgrounds to ensure variability and richness in the data. It might also incorporate high-resolution depth video data, allowing researchers to analyze the three-dimensional aspects of sign language that are vital for understanding and modeling. Furthermore, these datasets often come with detailed metadata and annotation layers that describe each sign, including its phonetic and morphological characteristics and contextual usage notes. This multi-layered approach enables a deep and multifaceted exploration of sign language, supporting various research and application purposes, from automated sign language recognition systems to educational tools for learning sign language.

Definition A sign language dataset is a specialized collection of data specifically designed to capture and represent the nuances of sign language communication. It typically includes video recordings of signers, annotated with detailed information about handshapes, movements, facial expressions, and body postures. These datasets are used to train machine learning models for sign language recognition and translation and to aid linguistic research into the structure and usage of sign languages.

Figure 7.1 presents a detailed illustration of the utilization and objectives of a sign language dataset. Initially, data is gathered from native signers or professional sign language interpreters [1]. This is followed by a critical data cleaning phase, which is essential for ensuring the accuracy and reliability of the data [2]. Once cleaned, this refined dataset becomes a valuable resource for applications such as sign language translation or synthesis [3], where it can be employed to enhance avatar technology, providing realistic and linguistically accurate sign language interpretations.

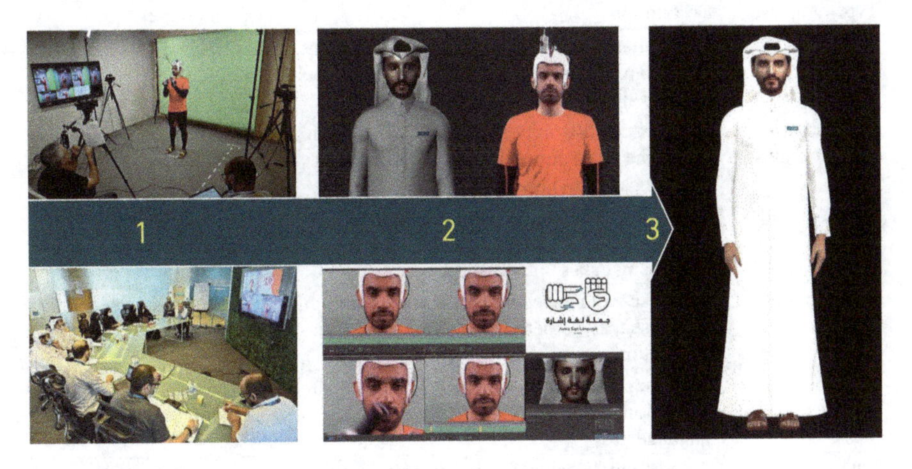

Fig. 7.1 Overview of sign language dataset construction and its usage

Sign language datasets are vital tools in the development of technologies for sign language recognition and translation, as well as for advancing academic research in sign linguistics. These datasets vary widely in type and scope, depending on their intended use, the depth of data they contain, and the technological approaches they support. Generally, the type of dataset selected for a project will significantly influence the outcomes of sign language processing applications, from educational tools to automated interpretation systems. Here, we categorize sign language datasets into several types, each designed to address specific research needs and application challenges. Here is a table summarizing the types of sign language datasets:

Each type of dataset has its unique characteristics and serves a different purpose, from supporting the development of technological solutions to enhancing the understanding of sign language structure and use.

7.3 Type of Sign Language Datasets

Table 7.1 provided an overview of the various types of sign language datasets, detailing their descriptions and typical uses. Each dataset category is tailored to support specific aspects of sign language processing and research, ranging from technological applications such as recognition and translation models to academic purposes, including linguistic analysis and kinematic studies. The table categorizes the datasets into six distinct types—Video-Based, 3D Motion Capture, Sensor-Based, Image-Based, Multimodal, and Linguistic—highlighting their primary characteristics and the typical applications for which they are most suited.

Table 7.1 Types of sign language datasets and their applications

Type of dataset	Description	Common uses
Video-Based Datasets	Collections of video recordings featuring signers using sign language, often annotated with labels for each sign.	Training sign recognition and translation models.
3D Motion Capture Datasets	Datasets that use motion capture technology to record the three-dimensional movements of a signer's hands and body.	Advanced research in sign language kinematics.
Sensor-Based Datasets	Utilize sensors (e.g., gloves equipped with sensors) to capture detailed motion and positioning data of hands and fingers.	Fine-grained analysis of hand shape and movement.
Image-Based Datasets	Comprise still images that capture specific signs or handshapes, sometimes used for static sign recognition.	Developing models that recognize individual signs.
Multimodal Datasets	Combine video, audio, and sometimes textual annotations to comprehensively view sign language use.	Multifaceted applications, including educational tools.
Linguistic Datasets	Heavily annotated with linguistic information, such as syntax, semantics, and phonological details of sign language.	Linguistic research and academic study of sign languages.

Video-Based Datasets

Video-based datasets are an integral resource in sign language research and technology development. These datasets typically consist of extensive collections of video recordings in which sign language users—comprising native signers or skilled interpreters—demonstrate a variety of signs and communicative gestures. The videos capture a wide range of linguistic elements, including handshapes, movements, facial expressions, and other non-manual features crucial for conveying meaning in sign languages.

Video-based datasets are characterized by their visual richness and temporal dynamics, offering a comprehensive view of the sign language communication process. Each video in these datasets is often annotated with labels that identify specific signs and their corresponding linguistic features. These annotations may include detailed descriptions of the context in which signs are used, phonetic details, and syntactic information, essential for linguistic analysis and training computational models in sign language processing.

Creating video-based datasets involves sophisticated recording equipment capable of capturing high-resolution images and maintaining frame integrity to depict the rapid movements involved in sign language accurately. Additionally, the recording environment is carefully controlled to ensure consistent lighting and minimal background distractions, which could interfere with the visual clarity of the sign language gestures.

Video-based datasets serve multiple purposes. Academically, they are invaluable for linguists studying sign language structure, usage, and evolution. These datasets enable researchers to perform detailed analyses of sign language grammar and lexicon, contributing to greater academic understanding and the development of comprehensive sign language dictionaries.

OpenASL and JUMLA-QSL-22 (Figs. 7.2 and 7.3) represent two significant contributions to sign language datasets, each serving unique purposes and addressing specific needs within the community of sign language research and technology development.

OpenASL is a publically accessible sign language dataset designed to support developing and testing automated sign language recognition systems [4]. This comprehensive dataset includes many ASL signs captured through high-quality video recordings. The videos in OpenASL feature a diverse group of signers from various backgrounds, ages, and regions, thus providing a rich source of data that reflects the natural variability in sign language use. Each video is meticulously annotated, not only with the signs being used but also with critical non-manual elements such as facial expressions and body posture, which are crucial for conveying grammatical and affective information in ASL.

JUMLA-QSL-22 is another innovative sign language dataset focusing specifically on Qatari Sign Language (QSL) [1]. Developed by the Mada Center in Qatar to address the lack of resources for QSL, this dataset is instrumental in promoting linguistic research and technological development for the Qatari Deaf community. Like OpenASL, JUMLA-QSL-22 includes high-quality videos of native QSL signers. These videos are annotated with precise linguistic details, offering insights into the unique characteristics of QSL.

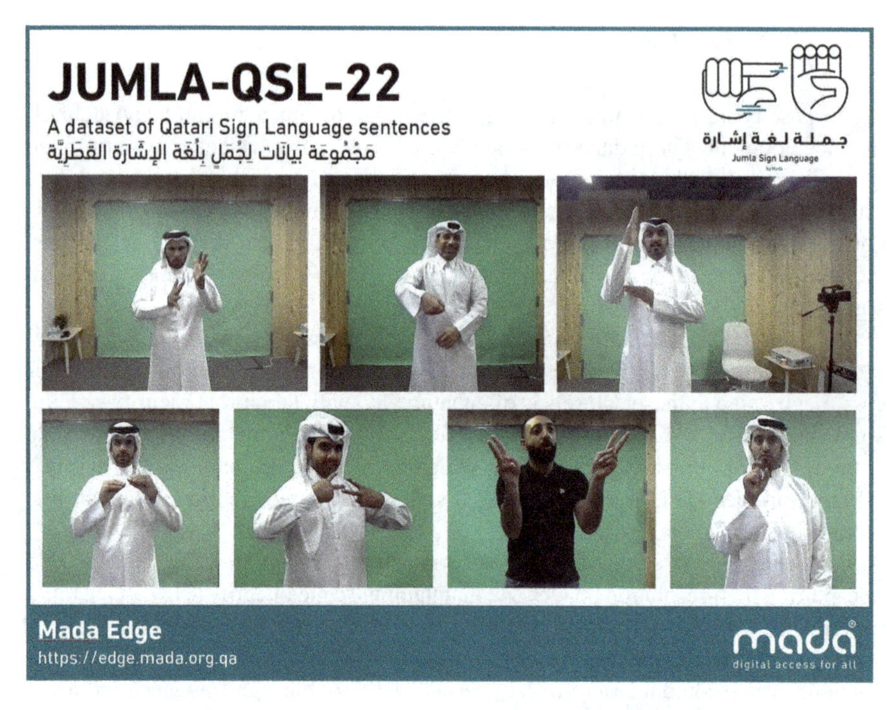

Fig. 7.2 JUMLA-QSL-22—a dataset of Qatari Sign Language Sentences

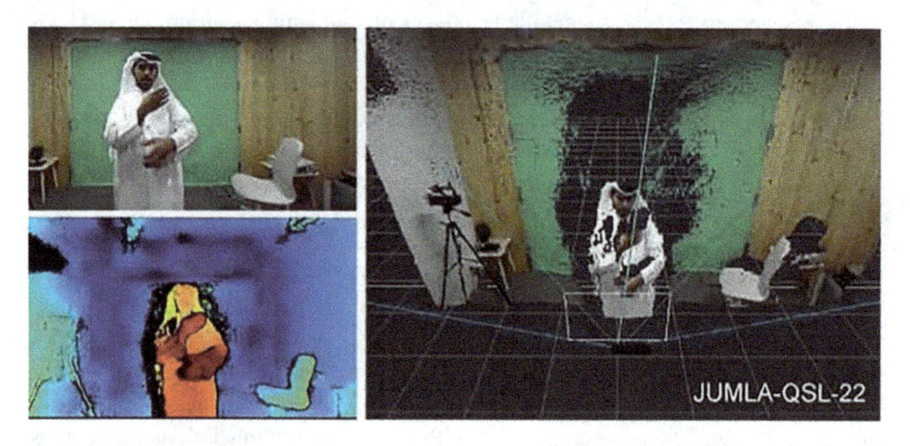

Fig. 7.3 Different types of video-based data collected during the recording (Raw RGB frame-based video, thermal data, 3D-depth data)

Beyond OpenASL and JUMLA-QSL-22, numerous other sign language datasets have been developed, each tailored to different sign languages worldwide. These datasets vary widely in scope and scale, encompassing a broad spectrum of regional and national sign languages such as BSL, JSL, and Brazilian Sign Language (Libras). Each dataset is designed to reflect its respective sign language's unique linguistic features and cultural nuances, providing essential resources for localized research and technology development. By capturing the diverse manifestations of sign language in various communities, these datasets facilitate the development of specific sign language recognition and translation systems and contribute to the broader understanding of sign linguistics and the promotion of cultural heritage within Deaf communities globally. The proliferation of these datasets underscores the growing recognition of the importance of accessibility and inclusivity in communication technologies, driving innovations that cater to the linguistic diversity of the global Deaf population.

A range of video-based sign language datasets have been developed, each with its unique focus. The American Sign Language Lexicon Video Dataset (ASLLVD) is a comprehensive resource for ASL signs, featuring linguistic annotations and verifications [5]. SignBD-Word is a dataset for Bangla sign language, including 2D body pose information [6]. The ASLLRP provides high-quality ASL video data, with manual and non-manual components annotated using SignStream®[1] [7]. The Word-Level American Sign Language (WLASL) dataset is a large-scale resource for ASL word recognition, with over 2000 words performed by 100 signers [8]. A dataset of hand gestures for emergencies in Indian sign language has also been developed [9]. The UWB-SL-Wild few-shot dataset is a training resource consisting of dictionary-scraped videos with class mappings to existing datasets [10]. Lastly, a video-based sign dictionary using linguistic sub-components has been developed, achieving high recognition rates [11].

3D Motion Capture Datasets

3D motion capture datasets represent a sophisticated branch of sign language resources that are pivotal for advancing the study and technological application of sign language. These datasets are generated through motion capture technology, which records the movements of sign language users in a three-dimensional space, providing a high-fidelity representation of dynamic gestures.

3D motion capture datasets are characterized by their ability to capture detailed kinematic data, including the precise positioning and velocity of hand movements, facial expressions, and overall body posture. This data is typically gathered using specialized equipment such as infrared cameras, reflective markers placed on the signer's hands and body, or inertial sensors that track movement through space without visual line-of-sight. The resulting datasets offer a granular view of sign language mechanics, capturing subtleties often lost in traditional two-dimensional video recordings.

The detailed kinematic and dynamic data provided by 3D motion capture datasets are invaluable for various applications. In academic research, these datasets

[1] About SignStream®: https://www.bu.edu/asllrp/SignStream/3/

enable linguists and cognitive scientists to analyze the physical mechanisms of sign language production and perception, contributing to language processing and development theories. For technology development, the precise data serve as a robust foundation for creating advanced sign language recognition systems, which can interpret nuanced signs more accurately than systems trained on less detailed datasets.

Despite their utility, 3D motion capture datasets are accompanied by several challenges. The setup required for capturing this data type is complex and costly, involving sophisticated equipment and controlled environments to ensure accuracy. Additionally, annotating these datasets is labor-intensive, requiring expert knowledge to accurately label the intricate movements captured in three dimensions. Furthermore, there are considerations related to the signer's comfort and naturalness of signing. The attachment of markers or sensors might inhibit natural movement, potentially altering the signer's usual gesture dynamics. Thus, researchers must carefully balance the need for detailed data capture with maintaining the ecological validity of the signing behavior.

Figure 7.4 depicts a motion capture setup for creating a 3D sign language dataset to capture the nuanced movements of sign language. In a studio environment, a subject wearing motion capture gear stands central in the frame, equipped with gloves and full-body sensors crucial for recording precise hand and body movements. To the subject's left and right, two tripod cameras are positioned to capture lateral movements, while a front camera, operated by an individual, captures a

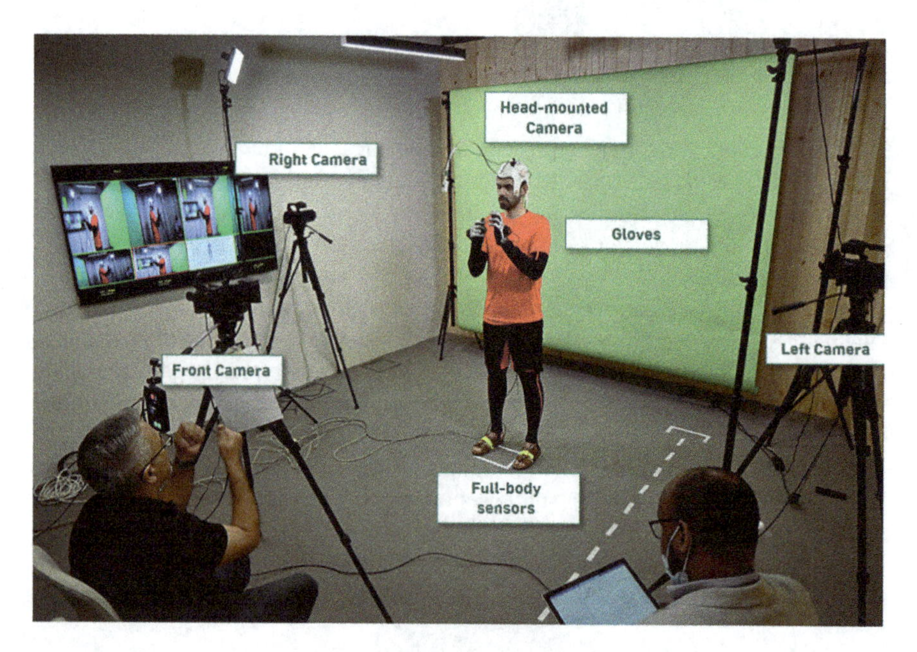

Fig. 7.4 An example of Studio setup to collect motion capture data to build sign language dataset (from [2])

head-on perspective. Above the subject is a head-mounted camera, presumably to gather detailed facial expressions, an essential component of sign language communication. The green screen background suggests the possibility of isolating the subject's movements from the background in post-production, allowing for a cleaner integration into digital environments. The presence of monitors in the background shows the real-time feed of the motion capture, enabling immediate feedback and adjustment. This setup exemplifies the comprehensive approach to producing high-quality 3D datasets for sign language research and technology development.

A range of 3D motion capture sign language datasets have been developed, each with its unique focus and contributions. Jedlička et al. present datasets for Czech Sign Language, with the latter being particularly large [12]. Kumar et al. and Watanabe et al. focus on Indian and Japanese sign languages respectively [13, 14]. Benchiheub et al. and Dibeklioglu et al. present datasets for French and Turkish sign languages respectively, using a stereo camera setup [15, 16]. Kiran et al. and Brock et al. explore using 3D motion capture data for sign language recognition, with the latter presenting a pipeline for generating 3D skeleton data from videos [17, 18].

Creating and using 3D motion capture datasets also raises ethical and privacy concerns. The detailed data can potentially be used to identify individuals, especially when facial expressions and body movements are captured alongside hand gestures. Researchers must adhere to strict ethical guidelines, ensuring that participants are fully informed and have consented to using their data in research and applications.

Sensor-Based Datasets

Sensor-based datasets for sign language constitute another facet of linguistic data collection. They leverage the latest in sensor technology to capture detailed motion and positioning data of sign language articulators—predominantly the hands and fingers. Unlike video-based datasets, which rely on visual capture of signing, sensor-based datasets utilize tactile and Inertial Measurement Units (IMUs) to provide granular data regarding the position, acceleration, and orientation of the signer's limbs in space.

The quintessential characteristic of sensor-based datasets is their high precision and granularity. Data gloves equipped with sensors, IMUs attached to the signer's arms and hands, and even head-mounted sensors to track facial expressions are some of the typical instruments used to generate these datasets. The sensors capture a wide array of data points in real-time, which are then translated into digital signals that precisely describe the sign language used.

An example of a sensor-based dataset is the EMG Arabic Sign Language Dataset collected using a Myo armband [19]. This dataset leverages the Myo armband's electromyography (EMG) sensors (Fig. 7.5), designed to detect electrical activity caused by skeletal muscle contractions. The armband, typically worn on the

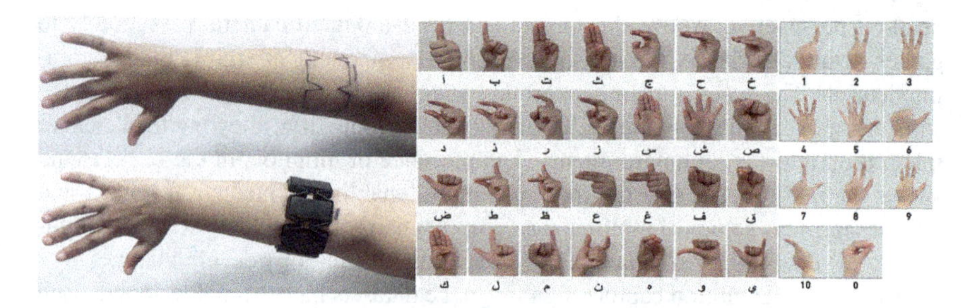

Fig. 7.5 An EMG Arabic sign language dataset collected from a Myo armband

forearm, is equipped with multiple EMG sensor pods that capture the intensity and patterns of muscle activity as different signs are executed.

During the collection process, participants wear the Myo armband while performing standardized sign language gestures. The armband captures the EMG data across its sensors, which is then synchronized and labeled corresponding to the specific signs being performed. The process is designed to be noninvasive and allow for the signer's natural flow of movement.

This dataset can be used to develop machine learning models capable of recognizing Arabic Sign Language from EMG data. These models can translate the EMG patterns into digital sign language representations or text, facilitating communication for Arabic Sign Language individuals. Moreover, because the data is based on muscle activity, the system can function in settings where visual sign language recognition is not feasible, such as when the signer's hands are not within the line of sight of a camera.

Image-Based Datasets

Image-based datasets serve as one of the foundational pillars in the repository of sign language resources, offering a static visual compendium of sign language gestures. These datasets typically comprise still images, each capturing a specific sign, gesture, or facial expression associated with sign language communication. Unlike video or motion-capture datasets, which encapsulate the dynamic flow of signing, image-based datasets focus on isolating individual signs or components, providing a snapshot in time.

The primary characteristic of image-based datasets is the encapsulation of discrete instances of sign language elements that are devoid of temporal context. Such datasets are constructed with meticulous attention to the clarity and definition of the images to ensure that each sign is visibly distinct and recognizable. This requires high-resolution imaging and controlled lighting conditions to prevent shadows and other visual distortions that could obscure hand shapes and facial expressions.

In sign language processing, image-based datasets are particularly valuable for training machine learning algorithms in sign recognition tasks. They provide a focused visual reference for each sign, which can be used to develop and refine algorithms for static sign recognition—essential for sign language technologies that rely on identifying individual signs without needing motion tracking or temporal analysis.

Creating an image-based sign language dataset involves a systematic photography and image editing approach. Each image must be consistently framed and annotated, often including a neutral background to prevent any distractions from the presented sign. Skilled signers or interpreters typically perform the signs to ensure accuracy and consistency across the dataset.

Image-based datasets are instrumental in applications where the static recognition of signs is required, such as in educational tools for learning sign language or in systems where users need to identify or practice individual signs. They also support research in computer vision and pattern recognition, contributing to the development of algorithms capable of recognizing signs from static images with high levels of accuracy.

Despite their utility, image-based datasets have limitations, particularly in conveying sign language's dynamic and contextual nature. Consequently, they are often supplemented with video-based or sensor-based datasets for comprehensive sign language recognition systems. The future of image-based datasets may involve integrating them with other forms of data to create multimodal resources that offer both the specificity of static images and the richness of dynamic data, facilitating more robust sign language recognition and translation technologies.

Multimodal Datasets

Multimodal datasets in sign language research encapsulate a comprehensive approach to data collection, integrating multiple streams of information to create a dataset that is both diverse in content and rich in context. These datasets typically combine video recordings, audio inputs, and sometimes kinesthetic data from sensor technologies, all synchronized to capture the full communicative intent of sign language.

Multimodal sign language datasets are characterized by their heterogeneous composition. They document the visual aspects of sign language through high-resolution videos and incorporate relevant auditory data, such as the signer's spoken words or environmental sounds that may impact the interpretation of signs. Additionally, sensor data can provide detailed information about the position and movement of the signer's limbs and, in some cases, haptic feedback, which can give insights into the physical interaction of the signer with their environment.

As an example from [20], authors presents an overview about the dataset. The How2Sign Multimodal dataset is an innovative sign language resource that is a testament to the multidimensional nature of sign language communication. This dataset is crafted to be a comprehensive tool for advancing research in sign language recognition and translation, and it is particularly notable for its integration of multiple modalities to capture the full spectrum of communicative cues used in sign language.

The amalgamation of data types in multimodal datasets facilitates a layered analysis of sign language. Researchers can dissect the interplay between visual gestures and spoken elements, examining how signers may simultaneously use spoken language, especially in bilingual contexts. The integration of different modalities allows for a deeper understanding of how various communicative signals are combined and perceived in naturalistic settings.

The acquisition and synchronization of multimodal data require an advanced technological framework. This often involves using multi-camera systems to capture different angles, microphones to record audio, and various sensors to track motion. The complexity of managing and aligning these data streams necessitates robust data processing and management systems to ensure the synchronization between modalities is maintained accurately throughout the dataset. In Fig. 7.6, the synchronization of different streams is implemented through controllers. This provides the accuracy of the annotation [2].

One of the primary challenges in creating multimodal datasets is the need for precise temporal alignment between modalities to ensure coherent data output. Additionally, the volume and variety of data present significant storage and processing demands. Ethical considerations also become more complex with multimodal datasets, as they often contain more personal information than single-modality datasets.

For sign language processing, multimodal datasets offer a foundation for developing sophisticated models capable of interpreting sign language holistically. They are crucial for advancing technologies such as automatic sign language translation,

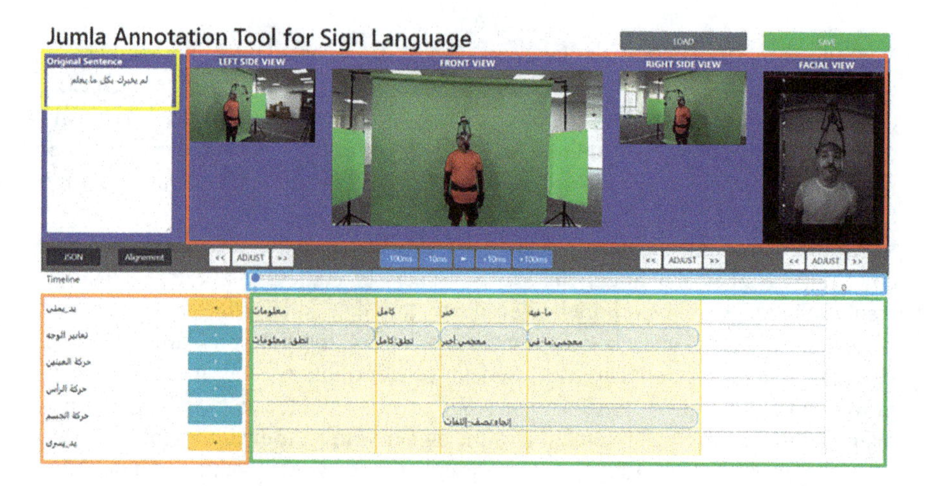

Fig. 7.6 A multimodal sign language dataset overview during the annotation task using gloss-notation system for Qatari Sign Language

where understanding the context is as important as recognizing the signs themselves. Moreover, they aid in creating immersive educational environments and virtual reality experiences where learners can engage with sign language on multiple sensory levels.

7.4 Building Sign Language Dataset Steps

As demonstrated in previous sections through different types of sign language datasets, building a sign language dataset is a multifaceted process that requires careful planning and execution. This section illustrates the different steps involved in constructing a sign language dataset and explains each step in detail details (Fig. 7.7).

Planning and Design

The initial stage involves outlining the objectives of the dataset and the specific requirements it needs to fulfill. Researchers must decide on the scope of the dataset, the sign languages to be included, the demographic representation of the signers, and the types of data to be collected. This phase also involves formulating ethical guidelines for data collection, including obtaining informed consent from all participants.

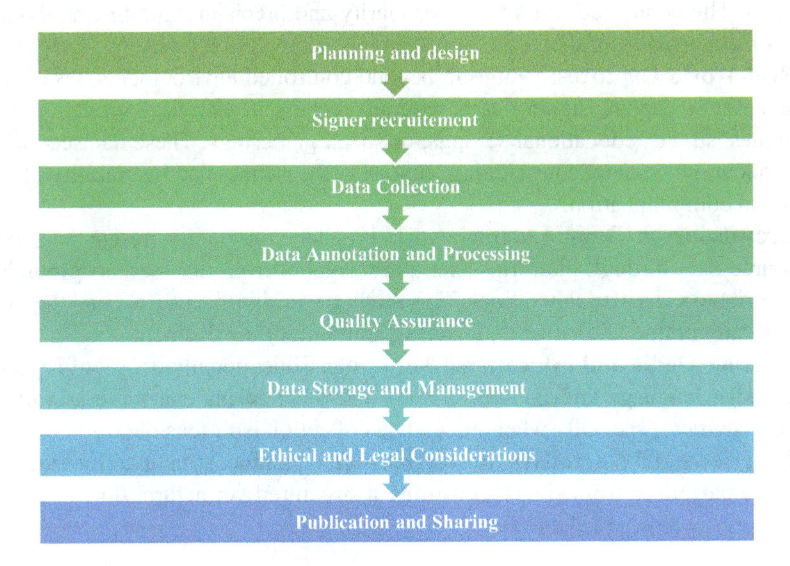

Fig. 7.7 Building sign language dataset steps

Signer Recruitment

A diverse group of signers is recruited to ensure that the dataset reflects a range of signing styles, regional variations, and demographic factors such as age, gender, and educational background. The recruitment process is conducted with cultural sensitivity and clear communication of the research goals and data usage policies.

Data Collection

This step involves the actual recording of sign language data. Depending on the dataset's design, data collection can include video recordings, motion capture data, sensor data, and audio recordings. The recording sessions are typically conducted in a controlled environment to ensure consistent lighting and sound quality, although some datasets may also include recordings from naturalistic settings.

Gathering accurate, comprehensive, and representative data is paramount to ensure that the ensuing research and technological advancements are authentic and effective. Data collection in the context of sign languages, with its inherent visual-spatial nuances, is a multifaceted effort, demanding both technological prowess and sensitivity to the signing community. Methods of Collection are:

- **Controlled Studio Recordings**: One of the most common methods involves recording signers in controlled environments, often studios equipped with high-definition cameras, proper lighting, and sometimes even motion-capture equipment. The controlled setting ensures clarity and precision, minimizing external distractions and variables.
- **Real-World Captures**: Venturing beyond controlled environments, researchers sometimes capture signing as it naturally occurs in everyday scenarios, be it homes, streets, educational settings, or social gatherings. These datasets offer a window into spontaneous signing, capturing the richness and variability of real-world communication.
- **Crowdsourced Data**: Leveraging the broader community, researchers often source data through platforms that allow signers from diverse backgrounds to contribute videos or annotations. This method can significantly expand the diversity and volume of data while fostering community involvement.
- **Existing Media and Educational Materials**: Educational videos, online tutorials, sign language television programs, and other media can serve as valuable data sources, especially when direct data collection isn't feasible.
- **Interviews and Narratives**: Researchers often conduct structured interviews or invite narratives from signers, ensuring a structured yet natural flow of signing on specific topics or themes.

Data Annotation and Processing

Once the raw data is collected, it must be annotated with linguistic information. This process may involve labeling the signs, describing non-manual features, and annotating the syntax and context of the signed communication. The annotation process requires sign language experts and often involves multiple rounds of review to ensure accuracy. Data processing also includes tasks such as video editing, audio synchronization, and the calibration of sensor data.

Quality Assurance

Quality checks are crucial to ensure the dataset's reliability and validity. This step may involve error checking in the annotations, reviewing the consistency of the recorded data, and verifying the alignment between different data types in multimodal datasets.

Data Storage and Management

Datasets, particularly multimodal ones, can be large and complex. Efficient data storage solutions and management systems are necessary to organize the data and facilitate easy access for future research. This step also encompasses implementing security measures to protect the privacy of the data subjects. Here are some mechanisms of storage:

- **Relational Databases**: These structured storage solutions often organize and store metadata, annotations, and links to visual resources. They allow for systematic categorization and easy retrieval, which is essential for extensive datasets.
- **Multimedia Repositories**: Given the visual nature of sign language data, specialized multimedia repositories become indispensable. These can store high-definition video recordings, motion capture data, and depth imagery, ensuring minimal loss of quality.
- **Cloud Storage Solutions**: The voluminous nature of visual data, especially when dealing with high-definition videos or motion capture sequences, often demands expansive storage spaces. Cloud solutions offer scalability, remote access, and frequently built-in tools for data management.
- **Local Storage**: While cloud solutions are becoming more prevalent, many research institutions still rely on local servers and storage networks, ensuring direct control over data access and security.

Ethical and Legal Considerations

Ethical and legal considerations must be at the forefront throughout the dataset-building process. This includes ensuring that data is collected, stored, and used in compliance with all relevant laws and regulations and the ethical guidelines established during the planning phase. Here are the main points to be taken into account:

- **Informed Consent**: Before recording, signers must be fully informed about the data's purpose, methodology, potential uses, and dissemination plans. Their participation should always be voluntary, with clear rights to withdraw.
- **Privacy**: Identifiable information, whether visual or contextual, should be protected and, if needed, anonymized to ensure signer privacy.
- **Cultural Sensitivity**: It is crucial to understand and respect the cultural, regional, and personal nuances of signers. This includes acknowledging regional variations and understanding that sign languages are deeply rooted in deaf culture and identity.
- **Compensation**: Given that signers contribute their time, expertise, and, often, personal narratives, appropriate compensation, whether monetary or kind, is fair and ethically correct.

Publication and Sharing

Finally, the dataset is prepared for publication and sharing with the broader research community. This may involve creating documentation to describe the dataset's structure, content, and instructions for use. It is also essential to decide on the terms of use, which govern how other researchers can access and use the dataset.

Each step is vital for creating a sign language dataset that is useful and respectful of the signing community. A well-constructed dataset has the potential to significantly advance the field of sign language research and the development of technologies that can facilitate communication for Deaf and hard-of-hearing individuals.

7.5 Conclusion

In concluding this chapter, we have comprehensively explored the various stages involved in building a sign language dataset. We began by understanding the critical role of datasets in linguistic and computational research, especially within the unique visual-spatial context of sign language. The subsequent sections provided a detailed road map of the dataset creation process, from the initial planning and design to the intricate data collection processes, annotation, and quality assurance.

We delved into the types of sign language datasets, such as video-based, 3D motion capture, sensor-based, image-based, and multimodal datasets, each offering distinct advantages and serving various research needs. This chapter emphasized the importance of considering dataset construction's cultural and ethical dimensions, highlighting the necessity of engaging with and respecting the Deaf community throughout the data collection process.

As we reflected on the diverse applications of these datasets in advancing sign language processing technologies, we acknowledged the challenges and responsibilities inherent in such endeavors. We examined best practices and innovative solutions shaping the future of sign language dataset development, ensuring that these resources foster academic and technological progress and enhance communication and accessibility for the Deaf community.

The journey through this chapter underscored the significance of meticulously curated datasets as cornerstones upon which the edifice of sign language technology is built. As researchers and technologists continue to refine and expand these datasets, we are reminded of their profound impact on bridging the communicative divide and enriching the lives of sign language users worldwide. With this foundation, we look forward to the continued growth and evolution of sign language processing and its boundless possibilities.

Quiz Time

1. What is the primary purpose of building sign language datasets?

(A) To collect data for educational purposes only
(B) To support linguistic research and the development of computational models
(C) To promote the sign language as a universal language

2. What unique challenges do sign language datasets face compared to spoken language datasets?

(A) They require less technological support
(B) They are based solely on textual data
(C) They must capture visual-spatial and often three-dimensional aspects of language

3. Which of the following is crucial for creating sign language datasets?

(A) Deep cultural and community engagement
(B) Focusing solely on the linguistic aspects without community input
(C) Limiting the datasets to video recordings only

4. What does the participatory approach in building sign language datasets emphasize?

(A) Engaging with community members as mere participants
(B) Engaging with community members as collaborators
(C) Excluding community feedback in the data collection process

5. What is an ethical consideration in building sign language datasets?

(A) Avoiding community involvement to speed up the process
(B) Ensuring that dataset creation respects cultural dimensions and community privacy
(C) Focusing only on technological advancements

6. What type of data do 3D motion capture sign language datasets typically capture?

(A) Audio recordings of sign language
(B) Detailed kinematic data, including precise positioning and velocity of hand movements
(C) Only static images of hand shapes

7. Which dataset is mentioned as focusing specifically on Qatari Sign Language?

(A) OpenASL
(B) JUMLA-QSL-22
(C) ASLLVD

8. What is the main focus of sensor-based datasets for sign language?

(A) Capturing audio variations in sign language
(B) Utilizing sensors to capture detailed motion and positioning data of hands and fingers
(C) Translating sign language into spoken language

9. What information is typically included in image-based sign language datasets?

(A) High-resolution audio files
(B) Still images capturing specific signs or handshapes
(C) Three-dimensional movement data

10. What role do multimodal datasets play in sign language research?

(A) They are limited to one type of data to simplify research
(B) They combine multiple types of data, such as video, audio, and sensor data, for a comprehensive analysis
(C) They exclusively focus on linguistic annotations without considering visual data

References

1. El Ghoul, O.E.G., Othman, A.O., Aziz, M.A., Sedrati, S.S.: JUMLA-QSL-22: A dataset of Qatari sign language sentences, https://ieee-dataport.org/open-access/jumla-qsl-22-dataset-qatari-sign-language-sentences. https://doi.org/10.21227/CKZP-3754.
2. Othman, A., El Ghoul, O., Aziz, M., Chemnad, K., Sedrati, S., Dhouib, A.: JUMLA-QSL-22: Creation and Annotation of a Qatari Sign Language Corpus for Sign Language Processing. In: Proceedings of the 16th International Conference on PErvasive Technologies Related to Assistive Environments. pp. 686–692 (2023).
3. Othman, A., El Ghoul, O.: BuHamad - The first Qatari virtual interpreter for Qatari Sign Language. NAFATH. 7, (2022). https://doi.org/10.54455/MCN.20.01.

4. Shi, B., Brentari, D., Shakhnarovich, G., Livescu, K.: Open-Domain Sign Language Translation Learned from Online Video, http://arxiv.org/abs/2205.12870, (2022).
5. Neidle, C., Thangali, A., Sclaroff, S.: Challenges in development of the American Sign Language Lexicon Video Dataset (ASLLVD) corpus. Presented at the (2012).
6. Sams, A., Akash, A.H., Rahman, S.M.M.: SignBD-Word: Video-Based Bangla Word-Level Sign Language and Pose Translation. In: 2023 14th International Conference on Computing Communication and Networking Technologies (ICCCNT). pp. 1–7. IEEE, Delhi, India (2023). https://doi.org/10.1109/ICCCNT56998.2023.10306914.
7. Neidle, C., Opoku, A., Metaxas, D.: ASL Video Corpora & Sign Bank: Resources Available through the American Sign Language Linguistic Research Project (ASLLRP), http://arxiv.org/abs/2201.07899, (2022).
8. Li, D., Opazo, C.R., Yu, X., Li, H.: Word-level Deep Sign Language Recognition from Video: A New Large-scale Dataset and Methods Comparison. In: 2020 IEEE Winter Conference on Applications of Computer Vision (WACV). pp. 1448–1458. IEEE, Snowmass Village, CO, USA (2020). https://doi.org/10.1109/WACV45572.2020.9093512.
9. Adithya, V., Rajesh, R.: Hand gestures for emergency situations: A video dataset based on words from Indian sign language. Data in Brief. 31, 106016 (2020). https://doi.org/10.1016/j.dib.2020.106016.
10. Bohacek, M., Hruz, M.: Learning from What is Already Out There: Few-shot Sign Language Recognition with Online Dictionaries. In: 2023 IEEE 17th International Conference on Automatic Face and Gesture Recognition (FG). pp. 1–6. IEEE, Waikoloa Beach, HI, USA (2023). https://doi.org/10.1109/FG57933.2023.10042544.
11. Cooper, H., Pugeault, N., Bowden, R.: Reading the signs: A video based sign dictionary. In: 2011 IEEE International Conference on Computer Vision Workshops (ICCV Workshops). pp. 914–919. IEEE, Barcelona, Spain (2011). https://doi.org/10.1109/ICCVW.2011.6130349.
12. Jedlička, P., Krňoul, Z., Železný, M., Muller, L.: MC-TRISLAN: A Large 3D Motion Capture Sign Language Data-set. Presented at the SIGNLANG (2022).
13. Kiran Kumar, E., Kishore, P.V.V., Sastry, A.S.C.S., Anil Kumar, D.: 3D Motion Capture for Indian Sign Language Recognition (SLR). In: Satapathy, S.C., Bhateja, V., and Das, S. (eds.) Smart Computing and Informatics. pp. 21–29. Springer Singapore, Singapore (2018). https://doi.org/10.1007/978-981-10-5547-8_3.
14. Watanabe, K., Nagashima, Y., Hara, D., Horiuchi, Y., Sako, S., Ichikawa, A.: Construction of a Japanese Sign Language Database with Various Data Types. In: Stephanidis, C. (ed.) HCI International 2019 - Posters. pp. 317–322. Springer International Publishing, Cham (2019). https://doi.org/10.1007/978-3-030-23522-2_41.
15. Benchiheub, M.-E.-F., Berret, B., Braffort, A.: Collecting and Analysing a Motion-Capture Corpus of French Sign Language. Presented at the (2016).
16. Dibeklioglu, H., Dikici, E., Santemiz, P., Balci, K., Akarun, L.: Sign Language Motion Tracking and Generating 3D Motion Pieces Using 2D Features. In: 2007 IEEE 15th Signal Processing and Communications Applications. pp. 1–4. IEEE, Eskisehir, Turkey (2007). https://doi.org/10.1109/SIU.2007.4298843.
17. Kiran, P.S., Kumar, D.A., Kishore, P.V.V., Kumar, E.K., Kumar, M.T.K., Sastry, A.S.C.S.: Investigation of 3-D Relational Geometric Features for Kernel-Based 3-D Sign Language Recognition. In: 2019 IEEE International Conference on Intelligent Systems and Green Technology (ICISGT). pp. 31–313. IEEE, Visakhapatnam, India (2019). https://doi.org/10.1109/ICISGT44072.2019.00022.
18. Brock, H., Law, F., Nakadai, K., Nagashima, Y.: Learning Three-dimensional Skeleton Data from Sign Language Video. ACM Trans. Intell. Syst. Technol. 11, 1–24 (2020). https://doi.org/10.1145/3377552.
19. Ben Haj Amor, A., El Ghoul, O., Jemni, M.: An EMG dataset for Arabic sign language alphabet letters and numbers. Data in Brief. 51, 109770 (2023). https://doi.org/10.1016/j.dib.2023.109770.
20. Duarte, A., Palaskar, S., Ventura, L., Ghadiyaram, D., DeHaan, K., Metze, F., Torres, J., Giro-i-Nieto, X.: How2Sign: A Large-scale Multimodal Dataset for Continuous American Sign Language, http://arxiv.org/abs/2008.08143, (2021).

Chapter 8
Sign Language Recognition

8.1 Introduction

Sign Language Recognition (SLR) represents a significant technological progression in artificial intelligence and computational linguistics. As defined in Chap. 6, SLR is "*the technological process by which sign language gestures are identified and interpreted through computational methods; they are then translated into text or spoken language to facilitate communication between deaf and hearing individuals*." SLR entails a series of complex processes to decode the rich tapestry of expressions and gestures that comprise sign languages.

SLR's fundamental objective is to render the visual-gestural mode of sign language comprehensible to non-sign language users, typically through spoken or written language. The technological challenge at hand pertains to detecting, monitoring, and classifying body postures, hand movements, and facial expressions. Sophisticated algorithms and high-resolution video processing are necessary for this purpose. In addition to accurately recognizing these signs, the ultimate objective of SLR systems is to comprehend their usage context, thereby guaranteeing an accurate translation.

The development of SLR commenced during the latter half of the twentieth century when initial undertakings were more concerned with deciphering isolated signs than conversational context or continuous signing. In the early stages of computing, computer algorithms primarily relied on colored markers or gloves to facilitate the detection of hand positions and movements. As technology progressed, researchers began to employ more naturalistic, markerless methodologies, enabled by advancements in computer vision and machine learning.

Significant transformations have occurred in the field of SLR over the last two decades, predominantly due to developments in deep learning. Antennas for Neural Networks (RNNs) and Convolutional Neural Networks (CNNs) have significantly transformed the ability to decipher intricate sign language sequences from video

A. Othman, *Sign Language Processing*,
https://doi.org/10.1007/978-3-031-68763-1_8

data directly. These models identify subtle nuances in sign language by acquiring knowledge from immense quantities of data, thereby substantially enhancing the precision and dependability of SLR systems.

SLR acts as a vital component in bridging communication gaps between the hearing and Deaf communities, thereby transcending the significance of the technological domain. SLR systems that function efficiently improve accessibility, specifically in education, media, and public services, enabling Deaf people to engage in conversations with greater autonomy and liberty in a society where spoken languages predominate. Furthermore, SLR can be life-saving in healthcare and emergencies by ensuring that Deaf individuals receive vital information without delay through real-time interpretation.

Furthermore, the integration of SLR technology into everyday devices, such as smartphones and tablets, can revolutionize communication methods for the Deaf community by providing instant access to translation services, thus fostering greater inclusion and participation in societal activities.

8.2 Foundational Concepts

Sign Language Recognition (SLR) is a complex and dynamic field at the intersection of computational linguistics, computer vision, and artificial intelligence. Its primary goal is to convert the gestural language of the Deaf community into spoken or written text, enhancing communication across different language modalities. According to the definition of SLR, this technological process involves capturing visual data, often through video, processing and analyzing that data to recognize and interpret signs, and translating these into written or spoken language. The accuracy and efficiency of SLR systems hinge on the recognition of several key components that constitute sign language:

- **Handshape**: The configuration of the hands during the sign. Different shapes correspond to different meanings.
- **Movement**: The action of the hands as they move from one position to another, which often includes the direction and speed of the movements.
- **Orientation**: The direction that the palms or fingers are facing during the sign which can change the meaning of the gesture.
- **Location**: Where the hands are positioned in relation to the signer's body, which can modify the sign's meaning.
- **Expression**: Non-manual elements such as facial expressions and body posture, which can convey crucial grammatical information and affective content.

The SLR process, as shown in Fig. 8.1, involves several steps, typically starting with data acquisition, where sign language interactions are captured using video recording devices. The data undergoes pre-processing to enhance image quality and segment the video into frames for more straightforward analysis.

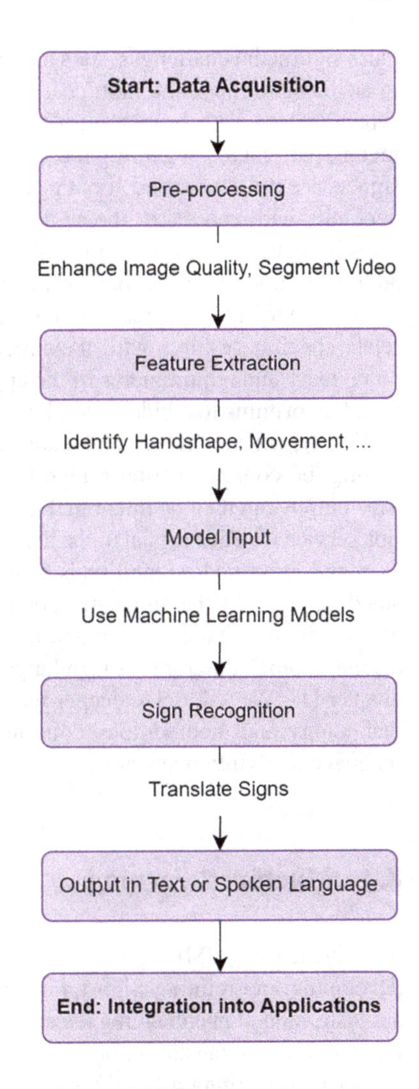

Fig. 8.1 Overview of SLR process

The next phase involves feature extraction, where critical information such as handshape, movement, orientation, location, and expression is identified using various image processing techniques. This stage is critical as the quality of the feature extraction directly impacts the recognition process's accuracy.

Data collection is pivotal and utilizes diverse techniques, each with challenges and ethical considerations. Video recording is the most common method, capturing a wide range of signs through high-resolution cameras. Motion capture systems offer more detailed data, tracing the precise movements of the signer's hands, face, and body, which can be critical for capturing subtle nuances of sign language. Sensor-based techniques involving equipment like data gloves or EMG sensors provide detailed data on hand positions and muscle movements, enhancing gesture recognition accuracy. Despite these technologies' benefits, data collection in SLR faces significant challenges, such as ensuring the naturalness of signers' movements in artificial settings, the high cost of advanced equipment, and the complexity of synchronizing data from multiple sources. Ethical considerations are also paramount, particularly regarding the privacy and consent of participants. Ensuring that signers are fully informed about how their data will be used and maintaining confidentiality and respect for the signers' cultural and linguistic identity are essential steps in SLR's ethical data collection. These challenges and ethical issues must be addressed thoughtfully to build effective and respectful SLR systems.

Once extracted features are input into machine learning models trained to correlate specific gestures with their meanings in sign language. Depending on the complexity and requirements of the application, these models can range from traditional algorithms like hidden Markov models to more advanced neural networks.

Finally, the recognized signs are translated into text or spoken language, completing the communication bridge from sign language to verbal or written forms. This output can then be integrated into various applications, from real-time translation services to educational tools, making them accessible to Deaf and hearing users.

Sign Language Recognition is a multifaceted process that requires a deep understanding of both the linguistic components of sign language and the technical aspects of pattern recognition and machine learning. Sharma et al.'s study presents a general block diagram for sign language recognition that will be discussed in this chapter [1]. We will delve deeper into these areas, exploring how advancements in technology and methodology continually enhance the efficacy and reach of sign language recognition systems.

8.3 Machine Learning

Machine learning (ML), particularly its subset deep learning, plays a central role in developing and refining Sign Language Recognition systems. These technologies are instrumental in enhancing the accuracy and efficiency of SLR by automating the recognition and translation of sign language into spoken or written language.

Machine learning algorithms enable computers to learn from and make predictions based on data, a feature crucial for recognizing the complex patterns of sign language. Deep learning, a more advanced machine learning, utilizes neural networks with multiple layers (deep networks) to analyze various data inputs. In the context of SLR, deep learning algorithms are particularly adept at processing the vast amounts of video data required for recognizing and interpreting sign language. They excel in identifying intricate patterns in data, such as the subtle differences in handshapes or facial expressions, which are often indistinguishable from less sophisticated algorithms [2].

The journey from traditional machine learning models to advanced neural networks in SLR reflects significant technological evolution. Initially, SLR systems relied on simpler models such as Hidden Markov Models (HMMs) [3] and Support Vector Machines (SVMs) [4]. These models effectively handled sequential data and classification tasks but often struggled with sign language's spatial and temporal complexities. As deep learning emerged, it brought the potential to overcome these limitations. Neural networks, especially Convolutional Neural Networks (CNNs) [5] and Recurrent Neural Networks (RNNs) [6], have proven particularly effective. CNNs excel in analyzing visual data, making them ideal for processing video images and extracting features such as hand position and movement. RNNs, on the other hand, handle sequential data more effectively, making them suitable for interpreting movements over time.

Table 8.1 from the study of Kasapbaşi et al. [7], showcases the accuracy of SLR algorithms using machine learning techniques. Methods achieved high accuracy.

Recent advances in machine learning architectures have further pushed the boundaries of what's possible in SLR. State-of-the-art models often include variations of CNNs and RNNs, such as LSTMs and Gated Recurrent Units (GRUs), which are adept at capturing long-range dependencies in data—crucial for understanding the context in sign language sequences. Additionally, Transformer models, which utilize self-attention mechanisms, are being adapted for SLR to better handle the alignment and translation tasks by focusing on relevant parts of the input sequences without the constraints of sequential processing.

Hybrid models that combine these architectures are also being explored to leverage the strengths of each. For example, a typical hybrid approach involves using CNNs to extract spatial features from video frames and an RNN or Transformer to interpret these features over time. This combination enables a more accurate and dynamic understanding of continuous sign language.

These advanced ML models require substantial computational resources and large, well-annotated datasets for training. As such, the development of SLR

Table 8.1 Comparison of the accuracy between different machine learning techniques (from [7])

Method	Accuracy
CNN [8]	92.88%
DNN [9]	90.3%
CNN/SVM [5]	98.581%/81.49%
PCAnet [10]	99.5%
ResNet-34 CNN [11]	78.5%
CNN and RNN [6]	93%
CNN-SVM [12]	98.30%
CNN [7]	99.38%

technology depends on algorithmic innovation and the availability of robust and diverse sign language data. The continued evolution of machine learning in SLR is a testament to the field's interdisciplinary nature, merging insights from linguistics, computer science, and engineering to build increasingly sophisticated and effective communication tools for the Deaf community.

8.4 Feature Extraction Techniques

Feature extraction is a critical component of Sign Language Recognition. It involves identifying and isolating meaningful information from raw data that is most relevant to understanding sign language. This step is crucial because the effectiveness of the subsequent recognition and translation processes heavily depends on the quality and relevance of the features extracted.

In the context of SLR, feature extraction typically involves processing video data to derive visual features that uniquely characterize sign language elements such as handshapes, movements, orientations, locations, and facial expressions. These features could be as simple as pixel intensity values or as complex as three-dimensional hand trajectories. Advanced techniques often seek to capture spatial features (like the shape and configuration of the hands) and temporal features (like the movement patterns over time). Techniques used include edge detection, motion detection, and optical flow calculations to analyze movement, as well as more sophisticated methods like depth sensing and three-dimensional reconstruction to understand the spatial dynamics of signing.

Feature extraction methods in SLR can be broadly categorized into manual and automated approaches. Manual feature extraction relies on human expertise to define features based on observable characteristics of sign language. These might include manually annotating images or videos with labels describing hand positions or facial expressions. While this method can benefit from human insight, especially in capturing subtle nuances of sign language, it is labor-intensive and potentially biased by the annotator's interpretation.

Automated feature extraction, on the other hand, utilizes algorithms to detect and extract features from data automatically. Techniques such as machine learning algorithms, particularly deep learning models like CNNs, are employed to learn feature representations directly from the data without explicit human intervention. Automated methods are generally more scalable and consistent, processing large datasets more efficiently than manual methods.

The quality of features extracted profoundly impacts the performance of SLR systems. High-quality features should capture the essential aspects of sign language that differentiate one sign from another and must be robust against variations in lighting, the signer's background, and clothing. Poor quality or irrelevant features can lead to misinterpretations and errors in the recognition phase, decreasing the overall accuracy and reliability of the SLR system.

Good feature extraction enhances the learning ability of machine learning models, leading to better generalization from training data to real-world usage. For instance, features that effectively capture the dynamic nature of sign language can help distinguish similar signs with subtle differences, significantly improving the system's precision.

8.5 Sign Language Recognition Algorithms

Sign Language Recognition algorithms form the core engine that drives the interpretation and translation of sign language into text or speech. These algorithms vary widely in their approaches, each with unique strengths and challenges, suited to different aspects of SLR. A detailed systematic review of SLR was done by Renjith et al. detailing all techniques used in SLR [13] and also presented previously in Table 8.1.

Hidden Markov Models (HMMs)

HMMs are statistical models that assume the modeled system is a Markov process with unobserved (hidden) states. In SLR, HMMs model the sequences of movements or gestures as a series of states, making them suitable for handling the temporal dynamics of sign language. The algorithm is often used for its ability to model time series data, where the recognition of a sign depends not only on the current state but also on previous states.

Convolutional Neural Networks (CNNs)

CNNs are deep learning algorithms that are particularly adept at processing data with a grid-like topology, such as images. For SLR, CNNs can extract robust spatial hierarchies of features through their layered architecture.

Recurrent Neural Networks (RNNs) and Long Short-Term Memory Networks (LSTMs)

RNNs are designed to handle sequential data, with LSTMs being a special kind of RNN capable of learning long-term dependencies. They are ideal for SLR because they can remember and utilize past information, which is crucial for continuous sign language recognition.

3D Convolutional Neural Networks (3D CNNs)

An extension of the traditional CNN that extracts features from both spatial and temporal dimensions, it analyzes video data in volumes. It is used to recognize actions in video sequences where understanding the movement across frames is necessary.

Transformer Models

Based on self-attention mechanisms, transformers analyze the entire data sequence at once, making them highly effective for parallel processing and capturing long-range dependencies.

8.6 Model Training and Evaluation

Training robust models for SLR and evaluating their effectiveness are critical components in developing accurate and reliable SLR systems. Various strategies are involved in model training, the key metrics used for model evaluation, and the best practices in dataset splitting to optimize training and testing phases. Here are some examples of strategies:

- **Data Augmentation**: Data augmentation techniques are essential to enhance the robustness of SLR models, especially in handling diverse signing styles and environmental conditions. These can include variations in lighting, background noise in videos, and artificial transformations applied to sign language videos, such as scaling, rotation, and cropping. Data augmentation helps in simulating a variety of signing scenarios, thus enabling the model to learn from a broader range of data instances.
- **Transfer Learning**: Transfer learning involves taking a model trained on a large dataset (usually in a related task or domain) and fine-tuning it to adapt to the specific requirements of SLR. This approach is particularly beneficial when the available sign language datasets are not large enough to train a deep learning model from scratch, providing a head start in learning general features.
- **Regularization Techniques**: To prevent overfitting, especially when training complex models on limited data, regularization techniques such as dropout, L2 regularization (adding a penalty on the size of the coefficients), and early stopping (halting training when performance on a validation set starts to deteriorate) are utilized. These techniques help develop models that generalize better to new, unseen data.
- **Ensemble Methods**: Combining predictions from multiple models can produce better results than any single model. Techniques such as bagging and boosting

Table 8.2 Evaluation metrics and validation methods in SLR

Metric/ method	Description
Accuracy	Measures the proportion of correct predictions made by the model out of the total number of cases evaluated. It is ideal for evenly distributed classes.
Precision	Assesses the accuracy of positive predictions, indicating the proportion of positive identifications that were actually correct.
Recall	This measure measures the model's ability to detect positive instances, representing the proportion of actual positives that were correctly identified.
F1-score	Combines precision and recall into a single metric by taking their harmonic mean, balancing the two when class distribution is uneven.
Confusion matrix	This provides a visual breakdown of the model's performance across different classes, showing where the model has confused one class for another.
Cross-validation	This involves splitting the dataset into multiple smaller sets that are used in rotating combinations to train and validate the model, maximizing the use of data and offering robust performance estimation.

can be employed to aggregate the strengths of various models, reducing the likelihood of errors that might occur from any one model's predictions.

In developing SLR models, dataset splitting is crucial in ensuring robust model performance. Typically, the dataset is divided into three key segments: about 70–80% is allocated for the training set, which is used to train the model and adjust the network's weights; around 10–15% is designated as the validation set, which aids in tuning the model's parameters and preventing overfitting by helping select the best hyperparameters; and the final 10–15% forms the testing set, used solely after the training and validation phases are complete. This testing set is an unbiased evaluator of the final model's performance, providing insights into how well the model will likely perform in real-world scenarios. Properly managing these segments ensures effective learning and validation, leading to more accurate and generalizable models.

A range of metrics and validation methods are employed to evaluate the performance of sign language recognition (SLR) models effectively. These tools are crucial for assessing the precision, reliability, and overall effectiveness of the models. Below is a detailed table outlining the various evaluation metrics and validation methods used in SLR, providing a concise overview of each method's focus and utility (Table 8.2).

8.7 Challenges in Sign Language Recognition

Sign Language Recognition (SLR) encapsulates many transformative possibilities for bridging communications between Deaf and hearing communities. However, the effective development and implementation of SLR systems are hindered by a variety of linguistic, technological, and data-related challenges.

Intrinsic Challenges of SLR

SLR systems must contend with considerable signer variability, where individual differences such as age, education, regional dialects, and personal signing styles impact the consistency of gesture recognition. Adding complexity, non-manual elements like facial expressions and body postures vary significantly among individuals, which are essential for conveying nuances in grammar and emotion. Context dependency also poses a significant challenge, as the meaning of signs can change based on the conversational context or surrounding signs, requiring SLR systems to process and understand sequences and their broader linguistic contexts.

Technological Hurdles in Real-Time Recognition

Real-time SLR demands high-speed processing to interpret and translate signs instantly. These systems face substantial computational demands, particularly when integrated into portable devices with limited processing power. Maintaining high accuracy and reliability in diverse environmental conditions—such as varying lighting and background disturbances—is crucial to avoid misinterpretations that could lead to significant consequences in critical applications.

Scarcity of Large-Scale, Annotated Datasets

The effectiveness of SLR heavily relies on access to extensive, well-annotated datasets, which are rare, especially for less common sign languages. Creating these resources requires significant investment, involving detailed collaboration with the Deaf community to ensure accurate representation and annotation. Additionally, ensuring diversity in these datasets is crucial for system effectiveness across various sign languages and dialects, presenting challenges not only in data collection but also in the comprehensive annotation of this data to capture a wide array of signing styles and cultural nuances.

8.8 Conclusion

In concluding this chapter on "Advancements in Sign Language Recognition," we have explored a broad spectrum of methodologies, technologies, and applications that underline the significant progress within this field. From the foundational aspects of sign language recognition to the nuanced complexities involved in machine learning models and the creation of robust recognition systems, this chapter has detailed the ongoing efforts to enhance communication capabilities between the Deaf and hearing communities.

The journey through this chapter has highlighted the critical role of sign language recognition in making educational and media content accessible, facilitating real-time communication, and ensuring that vital information reaches the Deaf community promptly. We have examined various SLR algorithms, noting their evolution from basic models to sophisticated neural networks that better capture sign language's dynamic and contextual nuances.

Moreover, we've discussed the challenges researchers and developers face, including the variability of sign language expressions among individuals, the technological demands of real-time recognition, and the scarcity of comprehensive, annotated datasets. Despite these challenges, the field continues to grow, driven by collaborative efforts between technologists, linguists, and the Deaf community, ensuring that the solutions developed are effective and respectful of cultural nuances.

As we look to the future, integrating SLR technologies into everyday devices and platforms promises to revolutionize how the Deaf community interacts with the world, breaking down long-standing barriers and fostering a more inclusive society. The advancements in SLR signify technological progress and reflect a broader commitment to accessibility and equality. This chapter has set the stage for further innovations and applications that will continue to enrich the lives of millions around the globe, making it an exciting time for researchers, practitioners, and users alike in sign language recognition.

Quiz Time

1. What is the primary goal of Sign Language Recognition (SLR)?

(A) To translate sign language into spoken languages to facilitate communication.
(B) To improve the quality of video transmissions.
(C) To create new sign languages.

2. Which technology has significantly transformed SLR capabilities in recent years?

(A) Neural Networks
(B) Fiber optics
(C) RFID technology

3. What is an example of early technology used in SLR systems?

(A) Colored markers or gloves
(B) Augmented reality
(C) Blockchain

4. What role do Convolutional Neural Networks (CNNs) play in SLR?

(A) They process audio inputs
(B) They analyze visual data and extract features
(C) They generate electricity

5. According to the chapter, what has been a critical factor in the evolution of SLR systems?

(A) Decrease in computing costs
(B) Advancements in machine learning
(C) Increase in manual processing

6. What is one application of SLR mentioned in the chapter?

(A) In automotive manufacturing
(B) In public services to improve accessibility
(C) In culinary arts

7. Which models are mentioned as enhancing the precision of SLR systems due to their ability to handle complex data sequences?

(A) Logistic Regression models
(B) Recurrent Neural Networks (RNNs)
(C) Linear Regression models

8. What is a challenge in SLR related to data collection?

(A) Ensuring the naturalness of signers' movements
(B) Reducing the color quality of video
(C) Increasing the speed of video recording

9. What is crucial for the ethical collection of data for SLR?

(A) Ignoring the privacy of participants
(B) Ensuring participant privacy and informed consent
(C) Collecting data without permission for quick results

10. How are modern SLR systems' operational capabilities described?

(A) Limited to offline use only
(B) Capable of real-time interpretation
(C) Only used in controlled laboratory settings

References

1. Sharma, S., Singh, S.: Recognition of Indian Sign Language (ISL) Using Deep Learning Model. Wireless Pers Commun. 123, 671–692 (2022). https://doi.org/10.1007/s11277-021-09152-1.
2. Adeyanju, I.A., Bello, O.O., Adegboye, M.A.: Machine learning methods for sign language recognition: A critical review and analysis. Intelligent Systems with Applications. 12, 200056 (2021). https://doi.org/10.1016/j.iswa.2021.200056.
3. Tornay, S., Aran, O., Magimai Doss, M.: An HMM Approach with Inherent Model Selection for Sign Language and Gesture Recognition. In: Calzolari, N., Béchet, F., Blache, P., Choukri, K., Cieri, C., Declerck, T., Goggi, S., Isahara, H., Maegaard, B., Mariani, J., Mazo, H., Moreno, A., Odijk, J., and Piperidis, S. (eds.) Proceedings of the Twelfth Language Resources

and Evaluation Conference. pp. 6049–6056. European Language Resources Association, Marseille, France (2020).
4. De Souza, C.R., Pizzolato, E.B.: Sign Language Recognition with Support Vector Machines and Hidden Conditional Random Fields: Going from Fingerspelling to Natural Articulated Words. In: Perner, P. (ed.) Machine Learning and Data Mining in Pattern Recognition. pp. 84–98. Springer Berlin Heidelberg, Berlin, Heidelberg (2013). https://doi.org/10.1007/978-3-642-39712-7_7.
5. Jain, V., Jain, A., Chauhan, A., Kotla, S.S., Gautam, A.: American Sign Language recognition using Support Vector Machine and Convolutional Neural Network. Int. J. Inf. Technol. 13, 1193–1200 (2021). https://doi.org/10.1007/s41870-021-00617-x.
6. Bantupalli, K., Xie, Y.: American Sign Language Recognition using Deep Learning and Computer Vision. In: 2018 IEEE International Conference on Big Data (Big Data). pp. 4896–4899. IEEE, Seattle, WA, USA (2018). https://doi.org/10.1109/BigData.2018.8622141.
7. Kasapbaşi, A., Elbushra, A.E.A., Al-Hardanee, O., Yilmaz, A.: DeepASLR: A CNN based human computer interface for American Sign Language recognition for hearing-impaired individuals. Computer Methods and Programs in Biomedicine Update. 2, 100048 (2022). https://doi.org/10.1016/j.cmpbup.2021.100048.
8. Rao, G.A., Syamala, K., Kishore, P.V.V., Sastry, A.S.C.S.: Deep convolutional neural networks for sign language recognition. In: 2018 Conference on Signal Processing And Communication Engineering Systems (SPACES). pp. 194–197. IEEE, Vijayawada (2018). https://doi.org/10.1109/SPACES.2018.8316344.
9. Daroya, R., Peralta, D., Naval, P.: Alphabet Sign Language Image Classification Using Deep Learning. In: TENCON 2018 - 2018 IEEE Region 10 Conference. pp. 0646–0650. IEEE, Jeju, Korea (South) (2018). 10.1109/TENCON.2018.8650241.
10. Aly, S., Osman, B., Aly, W., Saber, M.: Arabic sign language fingerspelling recognition from depth and intensity images. In: 2016 12th International Computer Engineering Conference (ICENCO). pp. 99–104. IEEE, Cairo, Egypt (2016). https://doi.org/10.1109/ICENCO.2016.7856452.
11. Kurhekar, P., Phadtare, J., Sinha, S., Shirsat, K.P.: Real Time Sign Language Estimation System. In: 2019 3rd International Conference on Trends in Electronics and Informatics (ICOEI). pp. 654–658. IEEE, Tirunelveli, India (2019). https://doi.org/10.1109/ICOEI.2019.8862701.
12. Nguyen, H.B.D., Do, H.N.: Deep Learning for American Sign Language Fingerspelling Recognition System. In: 2019 26th International Conference on Telecommunications (ICT). pp. 314–318. IEEE, Hanoi, Vietnam (2019). 10.1109/ICT.2019.8798856.
13. Renjith, S., Manazhy, R.: Sign language: a systematic review on classification and recognition. Multimed Tools Appl. (2024). https://doi.org/10.1007/s11042-024-18583-4.

Chapter 9
Sign Language Statistical Machine Translation: A Case Study

9.1 Introduction

Statistical Machine Translation (SMT) has long been recognized as a critical component of machine translation, having established the foundation for many language translations that have produced exceptional results [1]. By presenting unique challenges and opportunities, the integration of sign language offers a potentially fruitful avenue for improving communication between the deaf and hearing communities [2].

The present chapter investigates the application of Sign Language Statistical Machine Translation. This method integrates the complex visual-gestural characteristics of sign language with foreign languages' written or spoken forms.

The need for Sign Language SMT must be carefully evaluated. The Deaf community's access to information and communication heavily relies on the availability and accuracy of translation services. Implementing SMT for sign language aims to resolve this issue, facilitating effortless, dependable, and expeditious communication. This chapter will explore the nuances of tailoring SMT to sign language, explaining the specialized models, methods, and difficulties involved in this translation process.

The main goal of this chapter is to examine the use of sign language SMT, including its technological basis, model training, and refinement procedure, along with the practical factors that must be considered when utilizing these systems in real-life scenarios. This research seeks to provide a comprehensive analysis of the present condition of sign language SMT, emphasizing its current capabilities and prospective future developments that could significantly enhance the communication abilities of the deaf community.

A. Othman, *Sign Language Processing*,
https://doi.org/10.1007/978-3-031-68763-1_9

9.2 Foundational Concepts

The idea behind SMT is that translation processes can be modeled as statistical phenomena. Based on the probabilities of certain words and phrases occurring together, SMT systems learn how to translate text from one language to another. This section introduces the foundational concepts underlying SMT to better understand sign language's implementation.

Translation and language models are the two main components of SMT, which was initially developed for spoken and written languages. The Translation Model predicts the likelihood of a word or phrase in the source language being translated into the target language. Conversely, the Language Model assesses the grammatical and syntactic appropriateness of the text generated in the target language, ensuring that the output is accurate, contextually, and linguistically coherent.

The adaptation of these models involves unique challenges in sign language. Sign languages are inherently non-linear and use a multidimensional space to convey information through signs, which consist of combinations of hand shapes, orientations, movements, and facial expressions. These aspects necessitate adjustments to traditional SMT approaches, such as modifying alignment techniques to accommodate the visual-spatial nature of sign language and integrating non-manual features that play a grammatical role.

Figure 9.1 presents an example of a statistical machine translation applied to English and ASL from the work of Othman et al. [2]. Statistical machine translation requires two main models: language and translation. For hands-on implementation of a machine translation application between English and American Sign Language Gloss, please check the tutorial on my website.

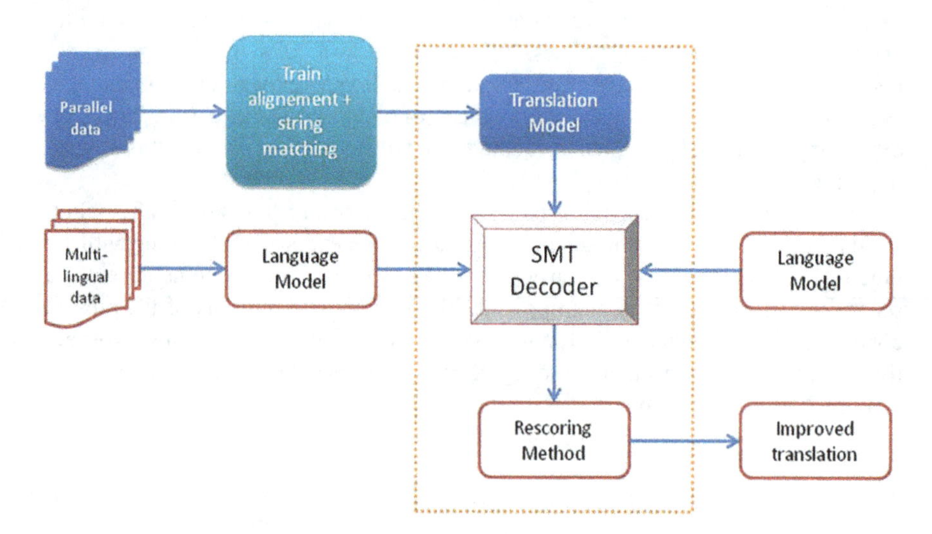

Fig. 9.1 Architecture of sign language SMT (from [2])

The historical development of SMT began with simple models based on word-for-word translation. It has evolved to incorporate more complex linguistic features and oversized context windows, greatly enhancing the quality of translations. The adaptation of SMT for sign language translation also follows this evolutionary path but requires innovative approaches to address the unique properties of sign languages.

9.3 Components of Sign Language SMT

SMT for sign language involves several critical components adapted to accommodate the unique characteristics of sign languages. Understanding these components is essential for developing effective translation systems to bridge the communication gap between sign language users and those who use spoken or written languages.

Translation Model

The translation model in sign language SMT is fundamental. It calculates the probabilities of translation equivalencies between the source sign language and the target spoken or written language. Due to the visual-spatial nature of sign languages, this model must handle lexical items and the spatial, kinetic, and gestural elements inherent in sign languages. This involves sophisticated algorithms that interpret and translate complex sign patterns into equivalent verbal expressions.

Language Model

The language model ensures that the output in the target language adheres to its grammatical and syntactic norms, providing translations that are not only accurate but also fluent. In the context of sign language SMT, special considerations must be made for modeling the target language, as the structure of sign language can significantly differ from that of spoken or written languages.

Alignment Model

Critical to sign language SMT, the alignment model maps the components of sign language—such as handshapes, movements, facial expressions, and their spatial orientations—to appropriate words or phrases in the target language. This component addresses the challenge of translating sign language's three-dimensional and gestural aspects into linear textual formats [3].

These foundational components work together to facilitate the translation from sign language to text. The translation model provides a dictionary of probable translations; the language model ensures these translations make sense in the target language, and the alignment model bridges the structural differences between sign language and spoken or written languages. Each component must be carefully developed and calibrated to handle the complexities of sign language, ensuring that the translation is possible, meaningful, and contextually appropriate.

9.4 Data Preparation and Processing

The effectiveness of Sign Language SMT heavily relies on the quality and preparation of the underlying data. Data preparation and processing are critical stages that involve several steps to ensure that the data used for training and testing the SMT models are well-suited for handling the unique aspects of sign language.

- **Data Collection Methods**: The first step in data preparation involves collecting a robust corpus of sign language data and corresponding translations in the target spoken or written language. This typically includes video recordings of sign language users, which must capture the manual signs and crucial non-manual elements like facial expressions and body postures. Parallel text data, where sign language video is annotated or subtitled in a target language, is essential for training effective translation models [4].
- **Corpus Requirements**: For SMT, the corpus must be large and representative, containing diverse examples of language use. This includes variations in dialects, signing style, and contextual usage to ensure the model can generalize well across real-world applications. The corpus should also be balanced, with a wide range of linguistic structures and vocabulary to cover the breadth of language typically encountered in everyday communication.
- **Data Cleaning and Preprocessing**: Once the data is collected, it must be cleaned and pre-processed. This includes removing corrupt or unusable data, normalizing data formats, and ensuring consistency across the dataset. In sign language, preprocessing might also involve segmenting continuous sign language footage into individual signs or phrases, which can then be aligned with their corresponding text in the training data.
- **Tokenization and Normalization of Sign Language Data**: Tokenization involves breaking down the video data into identifiable and discrete units of sign language that can be used as input to the SMT models. Normalization may involve standardizing the representation of these signs across the dataset to reduce variability irrelevant to the meaning of the signs, such as differences in signer positioning or background variations in the video data.

Each step is designed to enhance the data quality fed into the SMT system, which is crucial for the subsequent training of the translation and language models. Properly prepared data helps minimize the risk of introducing biases or errors into the SMT system and maximizes the performance and accuracy of the final translation outputs. The rigorous data preparation and processing phase lays a solid foundation for the effective deployment of sign language SMT systems, ensuring they are reliable and robust in practical applications.

9.5 Building the Translation Model

Building the translation model is pivotal to deploying a Sign Language SMT system. This model serves as the core mechanism by which the system translates sign language input into the target spoken or written language. The process involves several critical steps to ensure that the model translates accurately and maintains the original sign language's linguistic integrity and contextual relevance.

Training the SMT Model with Collected Data

Training the Sign Language SMT model with collected data is a foundational step that directly impacts the effectiveness and reliability of the translation system. This model development phase uses a specifically prepared dataset of examples of sign language expressions paired with accurate translations into a target spoken or written language.

- **Data Requirements and Preparation**: Before training can commence, the data used must be rigorously prepared and formatted appropriately. This typically involves collecting a large corpus of sign language videos, which must then be annotated with corresponding translations. Each sign language content must be accurately synchronized with its translation to ensure the model learns the correct associations. Additionally, the data should cover a broad spectrum of vocabulary, grammatical structures, and idiomatic expressions to train a model capable of handling diverse linguistic scenarios.
- **Model Learning Process**: The actual training process involves feeding this annotated data into the SMT model, allowing it to learn from the patterns and relationships in the data. The model uses statistical algorithms to determine the most likely translations for various sign language inputs based on the frequency and arrangement of signs and their corresponding textual translations in the training data. This process involves calculating probabilities that link sequences of signs with sequences of words, forming the basis for the model's translation predictions.

- **Iterative Optimization**: Training an SMT model is typically an iterative process, where the model's predictions are continuously compared against the correct translations. Discrepancies between the model's output and the actual translations serve as feedback, which adjusts the model's parameters. Techniques such as batch training, where the model is updated in increments as it processes subsets of the data, or online training, where each data point updates the model sequentially, are employed to enhance learning efficiency and model accuracy.
- **Evaluation and Adjustment**: Throughout the training phase, the model's performance is periodically evaluated using separate validation data that the model has not previously seen. This evaluation helps gauge how well the model generalizes beyond the training examples. Based on these evaluations, further adjustments might be made to the model's parameters or the training process, such as tweaking the learning rate, altering the model architecture, or introducing regularization strategies to prevent overfitting.
- **Balancing the Dataset**: Special attention is also given to the balance of the training data. Imbalances, where some signs or phrases are overrepresented, can lead to a model biased towards more frequent examples. Techniques such as undersampling the overrepresented classes or oversampling the underrepresented classes ensure a balanced training process accurately reflecting the diversity of sign language usage.

The meticulous training of the SMT model with carefully prepared and balanced data is crucial for developing a robust translation system. This trained model forms the heart of the SMT system, enabling it to perform reliable and accurate translations that can effectively facilitate communication between Deaf and hearing individuals in real-world applications.

Techniques for Parameter Estimation

Parameter estimation plays a critical role in developing SMT models for sign language, affecting the accuracy and fluency of translations. Techniques like expectation maximization (EM), Maximum Likelihood Estimation (MLE), Bayesian Estimation, and Good-Turing Discounting are central to refining these models.

- **Expectation-Maximization (EM)**: EM is pivotal for parameter estimation in models with latent variables, such as word alignments in SMT. The algorithm alternates between the Expectation step, which calculates expected log-likelihood based on current parameters, and the Maximization step, which updates parameters to maximize this likelihood. This method is beneficial in sign language SMT for iteratively refining the translation probabilities between sign sequences and corresponding textual phrases.
- **Maximum Likelihood Estimation (MLE)**: MLE determines parameters that make the observed translation data most probable. By defining a likelihood function based on the joint probability of the sign input and textual output, MLE

adjusts parameters to maximize this function, which is crucial for deriving accurate translation and language models in SMT.
- **Bayesian Estimation**: Incorporating prior knowledge about parameters, Bayesian estimation adjusts parameter estimates based on previous information and new data, producing a posterior distribution that reflects updated beliefs about parameter values. This approach is beneficial in sign language SMT, mainly when dealing with sparse data, as it allows for integrating prior linguistic insights into parameter estimation.
- **Good-Turing Discounting**: Addressing the zero-frequency problem where some potential translations do not appear in the training data, Good-Turing discounting reallocates probability mass from observed to unseen events. This smoothing technique is essential for language models in SMT, ensuring that the model can handle novel sign combinations not present in the training data.

Each technique contributes to building robust SMT models by ensuring that the parameters reflect both the training data and the inherent linguistic structures of sign language. Thus, the system's ability to deliver accurate and contextually appropriate translations is enhanced. These methods are integral to effectively translating sign language, facilitating more precise communication across language barriers.

Handling Data Sparsity

Data sparsity is a significant challenge in SMT, mainly when dealing with sign language, where the availability of large, annotated datasets is often limited [5]. This issue arises when there are insufficient examples of certain linguistic elements within the training data, leading to inadequate model learning and potentially poor translation performance for less common signs or phrases. To effectively handle data sparsity, several strategies and techniques are employed in the development of SMT models for sign language:

- **Smoothing Techniques**: These are employed to adjust the translation and language models so that rare occurrences do not overly influence the probability distribution. Techniques such as Laplace (add-one) smoothing, Good-Turing discounting, and Kneser-Ney smoothing are commonly used. These methods redistribute some probability mass from frequent to infrequent events, ensuring the model can handle unseen or rare sign-language input during translation tasks.
- **Back-off Models**: Back-off models provide a hierarchical approach to dealing with data sparsity by allowing the model to utilize lower-order n-grams when higher-order n-grams with the specific context are unavailable in the training data. This method ensures the model can still generate probable translations based on broader contexts when detailed examples are lacking.
- **Data Augmentation**: In sign language SMT, data augmentation can involve artificially creating new training examples through techniques such as synonym replacement, paraphrasing, or simulating variations in sign execution (such as

changes in signing speed or signer position). These methods help increase the volume and variety of training data, providing the model with a more prosperous learning environment.

- **Transfer Learning**: Leveraging models pre-trained on large datasets from related tasks or domains can also mitigate the effects of data sparsity. Transfer learning involves adapting these pre-trained models to the specific requirements of sign language translation. This approach allows the model to utilize learned features from a broader linguistic context, enhancing its performance even with sparse sign language data.
- Utilizing External Linguistic Resources: Incorporating external linguistic databases or lexicons can enrich the training data. For sign language, this might involve integrating databases of sign language dictionaries or corpora that provide additional examples and annotations. This integration helps to fill gaps in the training dataset, especially for rare or complex signs that require more nuanced understanding.

By implementing these strategies, SMT systems for sign language can better manage the challenges posed by data sparsity, leading to more robust and accurate translation models. These approaches ensure the translation system remains effective across various linguistic expressions, including those less commonly represented in the available training data.

General Note About the Translation Model

Building a robust translation model is a complex but critical task that requires a deep understanding of both the source sign language and the target spoken or written language. By meticulously training the model, fine-tuning its parameters, and ensuring it can handle the unique challenges of sign language translation, developers can create SMT systems that effectively bridge communication gaps between the Deaf and hearing communities. This process not only enhances the accessibility of various services and information for Deaf individuals but also contributes to the broader inclusion of sign languages in digital communication platforms.

9.6 Language Modeling for Sign Language

Language modeling for sign language in the SMT context encompasses complex and nuanced challenges and strategies. This process is crucial for ensuring that the output in the target spoken or written language maintains linguistic integrity and coherence. It involves developing robust models for these target languages and a deep understanding of sign language's unique structural and expressive elements.

Building Language Models for Target Spoken/ Written Languages

Developing effective language models for the target languages in SMT involves constructing statistical models that can predict the likelihood of a sequence of words. These models are typically based on analyzing large text corpora in the target language. The goal is to capture the linguistic patterns, syntax, and grammar that characterize natural language usage. N-gram models are commonly used, where the probability of each word occurring is conditioned on the occurrence of previous words in a sequence. This modeling ensures that the translated output is accurate in terms of meaning, fluent, and natural to the reader or listener.

Challenges in Modeling Sign Language Structure

Sign language presents unique modeling challenges because it fundamentally differs from spoken or written languages. Its grammar is three-dimensional and highly dependent on visual-spatial contexts, incorporating movements, handshapes, and orientations that do not have direct equivalents in spoken language. Additionally, sign language syntax allows simultaneous expressions conveying multiple grammatical elements simultaneously, a feature difficult to replicate in linear language models. These aspects require SMT systems to adopt more complex and flexible modeling approaches that accurately interpret and translate these multidimensional linguistic features.

Techniques for Integrating Non-manual Features

Non-manual features such as facial expressions and body postures play significant roles in sign language, often conveying essential grammatical information and affective content. Integrating these features into language models involves several advanced techniques:

- **Feature Extraction**: Advanced computer vision and machine learning techniques detect and classify non-manual features from video data. These features are then encoded as part of the input to the translation model.
- **Contextual and Sequential Analysis**: Techniques such as Hidden Markov Models (HMMs) and neural networks are employed to analyze the sequences in which non-manual features appear and their interaction with manual signs. This analysis helps in understanding the context and improving the accuracy of the translation.

- **Multi-modal Integration**: SMT models for sign language often need to be multi-modal, combining data from different sources (e.g., video, audio, and textual annotations) to fully capture the essence of sign language communication. This integration allows the model to use manual and non-manual cues to generate more accurate and contextually appropriate translations.

Overall, language modeling for sign language in SMT requires innovative approaches that go beyond traditional linguistic analysis. By effectively addressing the structural complexities of sign language and integrating crucial non-manual features, these models enhance the ability of SMT systems to deliver translations that are semantically accurate and rich in conveying the nuances inherent in sign language. This progress significantly contributes to breaking down communication barriers and fostering inclusivity for the Deaf community in a predominantly hearing world.

9.7 Decoding and Translation Generation

Decoding and translation generation are critical stages in the workflow of SMT systems, particularly for sign language. These processes involve the application of sophisticated algorithms to interpret the statistical models' output and generate accurate translations in the target language. Effective decoding ensures the translations are correct, contextually appropriate, and linguistically coherent.

Decoding Algorithms Used in SMT

According to the statistical models, decoding in SMT refers to finding the best target language translation given the source language input. This task is computationally intensive as it involves searching through many possible translations. Commonly used decoding algorithms include:

- **Beam Search**: This algorithm is widely used in SMT for its efficiency in finding the most probable translation. It limits the breadth of the search to only a few best options (the beam) at each step, significantly reducing the computational load while maintaining high-quality outputs.
- **Viterbi Algorithm**: Traditionally used in hidden Markov Models, the Viterbi algorithm finds the most likely sequence of hidden states. In the context of SMT, it helps determine the most likely sequence of words in the target language that corresponds to the sequence of signs in the source language.
- **Greedy Decoding**: This more straightforward approach selects the most likely word at each step in the translation process without considering future implications. While not as exhaustive as beam search, it is faster and can be effective in scenarios where computational resources are limited.

Strategies for Generating Accurate Translations

Generating accurate translations involves more than just literal word-to-word conversion; it requires the integration of linguistic and contextual nuances:

- **Language Model Integration**: During decoding, integrating a robust language model helps ensure that the translations are probable and grammatically and stylistically correct. This model assesses the fluency of potential translations and guides the decoder toward a more natural-sounding output.
- **Re-ranking**: A re-ranking step can be employed after the decoder generates initial hypotheses. Multiple translation candidates are scored and ranked based on additional criteria, such as length normalization or language model scores, to select the most appropriate translation.
- **Contextual Clues Utilization**: Effective decoders utilize contextual clues from the source data to make informed decisions about word choice and syntactic structure, which is particularly important in translating idiomatic expressions or culturally specific references.

Handling Ambiguities and Multiple Meaning Signs

Sign language has multiple meanings, depending on the context, facial expressions, and accompanying signs. Handling these ambiguities poses a significant challenge:

- **Disambiguation Techniques**: Advanced SMT systems employ disambiguation techniques to interpret signs with multiple meanings correctly. This may involve analyzing the broader context in which a sign appears or using statistical models to predict the most likely meaning based on surrounding signs.
- **Semantic Role Labeling**: Applying semantic role labeling can help understand each sign's function within a sentence, aiding in resolving ambiguities related to syntactic roles.
- **Feedback Mechanisms**: Implementing feedback mechanisms where the system can request clarification or additional context from the user when ambiguity is detected can significantly enhance the accuracy of the translation.

9.8 Evaluation of Sign Language SMT

Evaluating the performance of Sign Language SMT systems is essential to ensure their efficacy and usability in real-world scenarios. This evaluation involves a comprehensive blend of quantitative metrics and qualitative assessment methods alongside crucial user-based evaluations to incorporate feedback from the end-users, notably the Deaf community.

Metrics for Evaluating SMT Systems

Quantitative metrics are fundamental for assessing the accuracy and fluency of translations produced by SMT systems. These metrics provide objective data that can help in fine-tuning the systems:

- **BLEU (Bilingual Evaluation Understudy)**: BLEU is a widely used metric comparing machine-generated translations to one or more reference translations. BLEU scores are calculated based on the overlap of phrases between the translation and the reference, which are then weighted by a brevity penalty to discourage overly short translations [6].
- **METEOR (Metric for Evaluation of Translation with Explicit ORdering):**[1] METEOR extends beyond the n-gram matching used by BLEU by incorporating synonyms, stemming, and paraphrases. It aligns the translation and reference at the level of words and phrases, offering a more nuanced evaluation that accounts for meaning preservation and grammatical accuracy [7].
- **TER (Translation Edit Rate)**: TER measures the number of edits required to change a translation into one of the references. It provides insight into the extent of post-editing needed and helps evaluate the translation's efficiency from a post-editing standpoint [8].

Qualitative and Quantitative Assessment Methods

Beyond numerical scoring, qualitative assessments are crucial for understanding the contextual and cultural accuracy of translations:

- **Error Analysis**: This involves a detailed examination of the types of errors in a translation, such as linguistic inaccuracies, grammatical mistakes, or lost nuances. Error analysis helps identify specific areas where the SMT system needs improvement.
- **Contextual Evaluation**: Given the context-sensitive nature of sign language, it is essential to evaluate how well the SMT system handles idiomatic expressions, cultural references, and contextual cues. This often requires in-depth linguistic and cultural knowledge of the source and target languages.

[1] METEOR: https://www.cs.cmu.edu/~alavie/METEOR/

User-Based Evaluation: Involving the Deaf Community in the Testing Process

Involving the Deaf community in the evaluation process is vital for ensuring that the SMT system meets the practical needs of its users:

- **Usability Testing**: This involves members of the Deaf community using the SMT system in controlled tests to assess its usability, interface design, and overall user satisfaction. Feedback from these sessions is crucial for refining system design and functionality.
- **Real-World Testing**: Deploying the SMT system in real-world scenarios where Deaf individuals use it in their daily interactions can provide invaluable insights into its performance under varied and spontaneous conditions.
- **Community Feedback Sessions**: Organizing feedback sessions with the Deaf community can help gather qualitative insights on the translation's accuracy, cultural appropriateness, and emotional resonance.

Evaluating sign language SMT systems through these diverse methods ensures that they achieve high scores on standard metrics and are effective, user-friendly, and culturally respectful tools for the Deaf community. This comprehensive evaluation approach helps developers create more refined, sensitive, and accessible translation systems that effectively bridge communication gaps.

9.9 Deployment Challenges and Strategies

Deploying Sign Language SMT systems presents a unique set of challenges and requires strategic planning to ensure successful implementation. One of the primary hurdles is the technological requirement for processing complex sign language data in real time, which demands robust computational resources and highly optimized algorithms to achieve efficiency and speed. Ensuring the accuracy and reliability of translations in diverse real-world environments also poses significant challenges, particularly given the variability in individual sign language use, regional dialects, and the contextual nuances of sign communication. Moreover, integrating these systems into existing technological infrastructures, such as public service platforms, educational tools, or mobile applications, requires careful consideration of interface design and user interaction to accommodate the specific needs of Deaf users. Strategies to overcome these challenges include using advanced machine learning techniques such as deep learning for better performance and adaptability and developing modular system architectures that can be easily integrated into various platforms. Collaborative testing with the Deaf community is essential to refine system design and functionality, ensuring that the system is technologically sound, culturally sensitive, and user-friendly. Additionally, ongoing maintenance and updates are critical to adapting to language use changes over time and incorporating feedback from continuous user engagement. Effective deployment thus relies on a combination of technical excellence, thoughtful system design, and active community involvement to create translation tools that are both effective and empowering for the Deaf community.

9.10 Neural Machine Translation for Sign Language

Neural Machine Translation (NMT) represents a significant advancement in machine translation [9], offering substantial improvements over traditional statistical methods, particularly for translating sign language. Unlike statistical models that use fixed algorithms to translate text based on frequency and statistical likelihood, NMT utilizes deep learning to create a model that can more holistically learn the subtleties and complexities of language.

This approach is particularly beneficial for sign language as it can better handle the non-linear, multimodal aspects of sign language communication, such as simultaneous actions and facial expressions, which are crucial in conveying meaning. NMT models, typically based on Recurrent Neural Networks (RNNs), Convolutional Neural Networks (CNNs), or, more recently, transformer models, process sequential data and capture long-term dependencies more effectively, allowing for more nuanced understanding and generation of sign language translations [10–12].

Implementing NMT for sign language translation also involves overcoming specific data diversity and availability challenges. Due to its visual-spatial nature, sign language data is inherently more complex to capture and annotate than spoken or written language data. This complexity requires that NMT models be trained on large, well-annotated datasets that include a wide range of signs and contexts to improve the model's accuracy and generalizability. Furthermore, the training process must effectively incorporate the visual features of sign language, such as hand shapes, movements, and facial expressions, which are critical for accurate sign recognition and translation. Advanced techniques such as transfer learning are often employed to leverage existing datasets from related domains or languages, enhancing the NMT model's performance despite the challenges posed by limited sign language data.

The deployment of NMT systems for sign language not only enhances communication accessibility for the Deaf community but also opens up new avenues for academic research and practical applications. For example, NMT can facilitate real-time translation services that could be integrated into educational settings, public services, and media, making content more accessible to Deaf individuals. Moreover, the ongoing development and refinement of NMT models continue to push the boundaries of what is possible in sign language translation, promising ever more accurate and fluent translations.

9.11 Conclusion

In conclusion, this chapter thoroughly explores the complexities and innovative strategies of deploying Sign Language SMT. This detailed examination sheds light on the technical intricacies of adapting SMT for sign language and underscores its potential to enhance communication for the Deaf community significantly. Through a deep dive into various components, such as the translation and language models, the chapter highlights the necessity of sophisticated modeling techniques to handle the unique multimodal aspects of sign language. The discussions on data preparation and the challenges of model training illuminate the rigorous processes required to ensure that SMT systems are both practical and reliable.

Moreover, the chapter has critically addressed the deployment challenges, effectively suggesting robust strategies for integrating these complex systems into real-world applications. The engagement with the Deaf community during the testing phase emphasizes the importance of user-centered design and feedback in refining these technologies. By outlining future directions, including the integration of Neural Machine Translation (NMT) methodologies, the chapter reflects on current achievements and sets the stage for ongoing advancements that promise to push the boundaries of accessibility and functionality in communication technologies for the Deaf.

Quiz Time

1. What is Statistical Machine Translation's primary purpose for sign language?

(A) To improve the speed of sign language interpretation
(B) To enhance communication between the Deaf community and the hearing world
(C) To create new forms of sign languages

2. Which algorithm is widely used in SMT for finding the most probable translation?

(A) Linear Regression
(B) Beam Search
(C) Decision Trees

3. What is a critical challenge in modeling sign language structure for SMT?

(A) Its linear nature
(B) Its non-linear and visual-spatial nature
(C) Its reliance on verbal cues

4. Which method handles the zero-frequency problem in language modeling?

(A) Tokenization
(B) Good-Turing Discounting
(C) Neural Networking

5. What type of features are critical to integrate for accurate sign language recognition in SMT models?

(A) Textual features
(B) Non-manual features such as facial expressions and body posture
(C) Background noise features

6. Which technique helps estimate the parameters of an SMT model using both prior knowledge and observed data?

(A) Maximum Likelihood Estimation (MLE)
(B) Bayesian Estimation
(C) Linear Scaling

7. What is a common approach to mitigate data sparsity in SMT for sign language?

(A) Decreasing model complexity
(B) Data augmentation
(C) Reducing dataset size

8. Which evaluation metric aligns translation with reference at the level of words and phrases and accounts for synonyms, stemming, and paraphrases?

(A) BLEU
(B) METEOR
(C) TER

9. What does the alignment model do in the context of SMT?

(A) Maps gestures to appropriate phonetics
(B) Maps components of sign language to corresponding words or phrases in the target language
(C) Aligns audio with text transcription

10. What is crucial for an SMT system to effectively handle idiomatic expressions and cultural references?

(A) High-speed processing
(B) Contextual Clues Utilization
(C) Simplified translation algorithms

References

1. Koehn, P.: Statistical machine translation. Cambridge University Press, Cambridge; New York (2010).
2. Othman, A., Jemni, M.: Statistical Sign Language Machine Translation: from English written text to American Sign Language Gloss, http://arxiv.org/abs/1112.0168, (2011).
3. Bungeroth, J. and Ney, H., 2004, May. Statistical sign language translation. In sign-lang@ LREC 2004 (pp. 105-108). European Language Resources Association (ELRA).

4. Forster, J., Stein, D., Ormel, E., Crasborn, O., Ney, H.: Best Practice for Sign Language Data Collections Regarding the Needs of Data-Driven Recognition and Translation. In: Proceedings of the LREC2010 4th Workshop on the Representation and Processing of Sign Languages: Corpora and Sign Language Technologies. pp. 92–97. European Language Resources Association (ELRA), Valletta, Malta (2010).
5. Poulinakis, K., Drikakis, D., Kokkinakis, I.W., Spottswood, S.M.: Machine-Learning Methods on Noisy and Sparse Data. Mathematics. 11, 236 (2023). https://doi.org/10.3390/math11010236.
6. Papineni, K., Roukos, S., Ward, T., Zhu, W.-J.: BLEU: a method for automatic evaluation of machine translation. In: Proceedings of the 40th Annual Meeting on Association for Computational Linguistics. pp. 311–318. Association for Computational Linguistics, USA (2002). https://doi.org/10.3115/1073083.1073135.
7. Banerjee, S., Lavie, A.: METEOR: An Automatic Metric for MT Evaluation with Improved Correlation with Human Judgments. In: Goldstein, J., Lavie, A., Lin, C.-Y., and Voss, C. (eds.) Proceedings of the ACL Workshop on Intrinsic and Extrinsic Evaluation Measures for Machine Translation and/or Summarization. pp. 65–72. Association for Computational Linguistics, Ann Arbor, Michigan (2005).
8. Snover, M., Dorr, B., Schwartz, R., Micciulla, L., Makhoul, J.: A Study of Translation Edit Rate with Targeted Human Annotation. In: Proceedings of the 7th Conference of the Association for Machine Translation in the Americas: Technical Papers. pp. 223–231. Association for Machine Translation in the Americas, Cambridge, Massachusetts, USA (2006).
9. Koehn, P.: Neural machine translation. Cambridge University Press, New York (2020).
10. Lee, C.K.M., Ng, K.K.H., Chen, C.-H., Lau, H.C.W., Chung, S.Y., Tsoi, T.: American sign language recognition and training method with recurrent neural network. Expert Systems with Applications. 167, 114403 (2021). https://doi.org/10.1016/j.eswa.2020.114403.
11. Farooq, U., Mohd Rahim, M.S., Abid, A.: A multi-stack RNN-based neural machine translation model for English to Pakistan sign language translation. Neural Comput & Applic. 35, 13225–13238 (2023). https://doi.org/10.1007/s00521-023-08424-0.
12. Natarajan, B., Elakkiya, R., Prasad, M.L.: Sentence2SignGesture: a hybrid neural machine translation network for sign language video generation. J Ambient Intell Human Comput. 14, 9807–9821 (2023). https://doi.org/10.1007/s12652-021-03640-9.

Printed in the USA
CPSIA information can be obtained
at www.ICGtesting.com
CBHW070729160924
14542CB00003B/26